NO SWEAT

• • • • •

How the Simple Science of Motivation
Can Bring You a Lifetime of Fitness

• • • • •

MICHELLE SEGAR, Ph.D.

AMACOM

American Management Association
New York • Atlanta • Brussels • Chicago • Mexico City • San Francisco
Shanghai • Tokyo • Toronto • Washington, D.C.

Bulk discounts available. For details visit:
www.amacombooks.org/go/specialsales
Or contact special sales:
Phone: 800-250-5308
Email: specialsls@amanet.org
View all the AMACOM titles at: www.amacombooks.org
American Management Association: www.amanet.org

This publication is designed to provide accurate and authoritative information in regard to the subject matter covered. It is sold with the understanding that the publisher is not engaged in rendering legal, accounting, or other professional service. If legal advice or other expert assistance is required, the services of a competent professional person should be sought.

No Sweat is designed to provide helpful information on creating sustainable motivation and behavior change. This book does not make any medical recommendations and is not meant to be used to prevent or treat any medical condition.

LIBRARY OF CONGRESS CATALOGING-IN-PUBLICATION DATA
Segar, Michelle L.
  No sweat : how the simple science of motivation can bring you a lifetime of fitness / Michelle L. Segar. -- First Edition.
     pages cm
  Includes bibliographical references and index.
  ISBN 978-0-8144-3485-7 (pbk.) -- ISBN 978-0-8144-3486-4 (ebook) 1. Lifestyles. 2. Motivation (Psychology) 3. Self-care, Health. I. Title.
  HQ2042.S44 2015
  153.8--dc23
                               2014041322

About AMA
American Management Association (www.amanet.org) is a world leader in talent development, advancing the skills of individuals to drive business success. Our mission is to support the goals of individuals and organizations through a complete range of products and services, including classroom and virtual seminars, webcasts, webinars, podcasts, conferences, corporate and government solutions, business books, and research. AMA's approach to improving performance combines experiential learning—learning through doing—with opportunities for ongoing professional growth at every step of one's career journey.

Printing number
10 9 8 7 6 5 4 3 2 1

"Dr. Michelle Segar has pioneered solutions for sustainable behavior change that are being used within organizational wellness and health care settings. We are excited to be applying her insights to help large organizations move into the new frontier of organizational well-being."
    —LuAnn Heinen, Vice President, National Business Group on Health

"Dr. Segar's book can be used by clinicians and patients alike as an inspiring new tool to engage people in prioritizing their own self-care and sustaining their lifestyle goals with enthusiasm and energy."
    —Rita Antonson, MSN, APRN, GNP-BC, University of Nebraska Medical Center, College of Nursing

"Forget all the reasons why you think you *should* exercise! In *No Sweat*, Dr. Segar makes a compelling case for a new approach to how we relate to physical activity. Balancing her experience as both a researcher and an exercise counsellor, and drawing on the most advanced science on behavior change, she offers a much-needed guide to both health professionals and the general public. If physical activity is to be a success story in public health and have a lasting impact on people's lives, we urgently need to a change in perspective. Dr. Segar shows how we can move toward that goal, by understanding how long-lasting motivation is nurtured, focusing on self-awareness and self-care, and using self-regulatory skills that effectively sustain a more active lifestyle."
    —Pedro Teixeira, Ph.D., Past President, International Society of Behavioral Nutrition and Physical Activity; and Director of the Physical Activity, Nutrition, and Obesity Group at the University of Lisbon, Portugal

"As a personal trainer for 20 years, I have learned that no exercise regimen will work, regardless of intention, without being intrinsically motivated. In *No Sweat*, Michelle Segar gives fitness professionals like me a detailed and easy-to-understand method to help clients develop a personalized 'roadmap' to making lasting changes and a healthier lifestyle."
    —Dawn Lovejoy, certified personal trainer, YMCA of Central Massachusetts, Worcester, Massachusetts

"*No Sweat* reminds us that counseling methods based on motivation psychology and decision making are more impactful than imploring health-promoting behavior change with our patients who need to make lifestyle modifications. Using real client stories and research, Segar shows us how to get better behavioral outcomes with patients, using an incremental strategy. This book will be valuable for individuals trying to make fitness changes on their own, and for physicians who need patient aids to encourage lifestyle modifications."

—Halley S. Faust, M.D., MPH, MA, Past President, American College of Preventive Medicine; and Clinical Associate Professor, Department of Family and Community Medicine, University of New Mexico

"In this exceptional, evidence-based book, Michelle Segar shows us how to make truly lasting changes in our own lives and in the lives of others. It will be a centrally important book for both wellness coaches and their clients."

—Ben Dean, Ph.D., Founder, MentorCoach; co-author, *Positive Psychology Coaching*

To my mom and dad and my love, Jeff,
for inspiring me to be the best I can be
and supporting me every step of the way,
and to Eli, the greatest gift of all.

Contents

Contents

PART III.
PERMISSION

PART IV.
STRATEGY

Contents

List of Figures

Preface

I LIVE IN ANN ARBOR, MICHIGAN, WITH MY HUSBAND AND SEVEN-YEAR-old son in a house we chose because it was close enough to town that we could do errands and get to work on foot or bike. Yes, I'm in good physical condition, but I am not one of those people who spends every morning at the gym or goes around spouting platitudes like "No pain, no gain." In fact, growing up I was always a little awkward, a little shy, and not the girl who was picked first (or second or third) for most team sports.

Then, when I entered puberty, my self-esteem plummeted. One day after school, when I was at odds with myself and the world, I decided to put on my sneakers and jog around the neighborhood. I was probably out for only about fifteen minutes, but the effect on my mood was profound. At that moment something within me clicked. From then on I understood that when I was feeling low, getting outdoors and moving would help.

Did I go on to become an elite runner? No. Although I've always enjoyed running, I really love to walk. I rely on walking not only to nourish my body but also to clear my mind.

I did, however, decide to spend my professional life studying what motivates people to get off the couch and go out running, walking, or engaging in whatever sort of physical activity they prefer or want to do in the moment so they stick with it through life. My interdisciplinary research challenges the status quo within the health promotion and healthcare industries by showing that logical rewards like "health" and "weight loss" do not motivate people to sustain health-related behavior as well as immediate and emotional rewards such as "well-being." These findings have propelled me to create game-changing wellness systems, protocols, and messages that motivate individuals to prioritize and sustain physically active lives and other positive health behaviors.

These provocative ideas have gained the attention of both the media and influential members of the health field. I am widely quoted in the media and consulted as an expert by major publications like the *New York Times* and government agencies like the U.S. Department of Health and Human Services. My evidence-based ideas have generated accolades from such prestigious organizations as the Society of Behavioral Medicine, the Blue Cross Blue Shield of Michigan Foundation, and the North American Menopause Society, among many others.

I am passionately devoted to the science of motivation. I chose to get my doctorate in the Personality area of the Psychology Department at the University of Michigan because this is where the field of motivation originated. I was eager to develop a deep understanding of how to create sustainable motivation, goal pursuit, and behavior, and I learned many important things during this time.

But one particular thing I learned grabbed onto me and wouldn't let me go: Despite the pioneering findings showing that motivation is inextricably connected to our personality and to the "self," in today's typical conversations about promoting healthy lifestyles and self-care behaviors, professionals rarely talk about the self. Yet the secret to achieving sustainable self-perpetual behavior change lies precisely in understanding how to create goals, motivation, and behavior that reflect what is most aligned with and meaningful to our sense of self.

I love my work, and I love helping others learn how they can use natural, human movement to get happy, stay healthy, and become energized for a lifetime. Some of my clients were gracious enough to allow me to share their stories and comments in this book. I have done so gratefully, changing their names in all cases. Some stories are composites, but the details are true to experience. My clients are also my teachers. I learn something new from them every day, and I am delighted to share this with you.

There is a mountain of information out there about health and fitness, but most of it is just not working for people. I wrote this book to help you understand the science-based reasons why it's *not your fault* that you've failed to stick with exercise and other health-related behaviors, as well as to give you a new, simple framework for sustainable success. Opportunities to move and enjoy physical movement are, quite literally, everywhere. I hope that the information and practical approaches in this book will enable you to find them, choose them, enjoy them, and use them to energize your life for a lifetime.

Acknowledgments

NO SWEAT REPRESENTS AN INTEGRATION OF THE EXPERIENCES, research, and training I've had over the last twenty-one years, so there are many people I want to thank. I have learned from and been inspired by many scholars, clients, business professionals, family members, and friends. Everyone, combined, has played a role in forming the gestalt of my thinking and helping me take a simple insight from research and translate it into a real-life solution that helps people feel better and energizes them to sustain happier and healthier lives. It has been a true labor of love.

First and foremost, I am grateful to Naomi Lucks for the invaluable editorial insights she brought to *No Sweat*. I am also thankful to Robert Nirkind and AMACOM Books for believing in my comprehensive system and the need to get it out into the world. Another special thank you goes to my agent, Lauren Galit, who guided and advised me throughout the entire book process.

The integration of ideas in *No Sweat* is uniquely mine, but these ideas stand on the shoulders of the research and work of many insightful scholars. The following thinkers greatly influenced my foundational ideas about how to develop systems for sustainable behavior change that simultaneously fuel people to live happier, more fulfilling lives: Gordon Allport, Richard Bagozzi, Kent Berridge,

Charles Carver and Michael Scheier, Robert Cialdini, Richard Davidson, Edward Deci and Richard Ryan, Carol Dweck, Jacquelynne Eccles, Panteleimon Ekkekakis, Seymour Epstein, Barbara Fredrickson, Paulo Freire, Winifred Gebhardt, Peter Gollwitzer, Karla Henderson, Wilhelm Hofmann and Reinout Wiers, Jon Kabat-Zinn, Paul Karoly, George Kelly, Julius Kuhl, Richard Lazarus, Howard Leventhal, Brian Little, Carol Ryff, and Ken Sheldon.

I am also grateful to those who have mentored and supported me. First and foremost, I want to thank the person without whose mentorship and encouragement I would not have discovered my professional passion and purpose: Vic Katch. Vic, thanks for being a great teacher, igniting my love of research, and giving me my wings (in addition to guiding me right to my husband and copilot, Jeff). Others who have been guides and/or supports at key points on my path include Doris Aaron, Jesse Bernstein, Carol Boyd, Chris Bidlack and Jeannette Gutierrez, Kathy Caprino, Noreen Clark, Julie Dodge, Jacquelynne Eccles, Nancy Janz, Jayme Johnson, Jennifer Martin, Susan Nolen-Hoeksema, Chris Peterson, Caroline Richardson, Randy Roth, Joan Hallem Schafer, and Peter Ubel.

I am thankful to the University of Michigan for training me to be a critical thinker, cultivating my curiosity, and quenching my thirst for actionable knowledge. I am also especially grateful to all of my clients for trusting me to be their guide for the last two decades and teaching me so much along the way.

A tremendous thank you goes to my dear friends and family for always being there and tolerating many intense conversations about the key principles of my work. I am forever grateful to my husband, Jeff Horowitz, and our son, Eli, who encourage me to follow my dream even though it takes me away sometimes. I love you both more than words can say. Finally, I want to thank my mom and dad, Ilene and Bob Segar, for encouraging me to forge my own path and supporting me every step of the way.

A Note to Health and Wellness Professionals

IF YOU READ THIS BOOK, YOU ARE LIKELY INTERESTED IN BETTER understanding why so many of your patients fail to stick with their intentions to exercise, change their eating habits, and lose weight—and what you can do to change this. This book was designed to help you in your professional capacity as well as in your own life.

As you've seen in your work, getting people to say they want to change their health behaviors can come easily—at first. The problem is that people quickly revert to old habits, resulting in high rates of disease, lost productivity, poor mental health, and spiraling health-care costs. Most of us in health promotion and healthcare have been taught that we should promote "better health" and "disease prevention" as the valuable outcomes to motivate people to practice the life-style behaviors necessary for healthier living and disease management.

The problem is that what we've learned and how we've been taught to prescribe "behavior" comes out of a medical framework, one that doesn't take human decision making, motivation, and behavior into account.

Research shows that future health benefits, such as disease prevention, are too abstract to overcome people's inertia and hectic schedules. When motivation is linked to distant, clinical, or abstract goals, health behaviors are not compelling enough to trump the many other daily goals and priorities they constantly compete with. Even weight loss as an impetus for diet and exercise, particularly for women, is often based in self-rejection; while it is great at eliciting intentions to change, in the long run it frequently fails to motivate behavior long term.

In this new era of healthcare, patient self-management and self-regulation decisions are essential for improving outcomes and decreasing costs. Yet, as a result of the many distractions and alternative choices that are a constant part of their busy daily lives, patients are at risk of self-management failure. A prescription for lifestyle change to optimize health seems like good medicine. But if most people are not motivated to sustain it over time, then the actual health benefits will be small.

In fact, we might even consider that promoting the wrong reasons for a behavior change as being a very costly strategy, expensive for everyone. It's expensive for our organizations because they are investing their resources in promoting future reasons for change that tend to drive short-term results (not a very good ROI). It's expensive for us professionals because when the people we counsel don't follow through we feel discouraged and ineffective, and maybe even stop enjoying our work (a recipe for burnout). It's expensive for our patients and clients because they *really do* want to change, so when they are not successful sustaining their desired behavioral changes, their hopes are dashed and they often become ambivalent about and resistant to investing again in their own self-care.

The health-related reasons for making lifestyle changes that we health professionals care about are irrelevant to which reasons will be most relevant and compelling to patients' lives. It doesn't matter whether or not things like weight loss or better health are "good" or actual goals that we want our patients to achieve from behaviors like physical activity. It does matter, however, that these goals may be ineffective for many because they don't make physical activity explicitly relevant to our most important daily roles and priorities. As a result, these types of goals don't imbue exercising with the type of significance that has the positivity and potency to *consistently* motivate most people to prioritize and sustain physical activity and other self-care behaviors in their lives. My research and other science suggest that people are more likely to sustain behaviors that are essential to their daily lives *in immediate and noticeable ways.** This simple idea is also supported by the tried and true methods that marketers use to promote ongoing customer behavior.

No Sweat is written for individuals looking for real and sustainable ways to feel better, live better, and become happier, healthier, and fit. Because most people who intend to get healthy or who start exercising drop out within six months, professionals who work with patients, businesses that promote exercise to their employees, and the government, which funds Medicaid and Medicare, are all desperate for new behavioral solutions that are grounded in research and that can actually work long term.

No Sweat provides a scientifically supported, simple, and time-tested health-and-fitness solution that can fill this need for a very large market. *However, the approach I teach should not replace medically necessary behaviors.* My approach, though, can be used as a strategic ally— as an "in"—to enhance motivation even when there is a very real and compelling medical need. This philosophy and approach is inherently patient-centered. I hope *No Sweat* can help you identify new ways to help your patients discover the reasons that will truly motivate them, and that you will recommend the book to your clients and patients, especially those who are ambivalent or lack the motivation to stick with self-care behaviors, like physical activity, sleep, or dietary changes for the long term. *No Sweat* is also a resource for people who don't feel comfortable or confident prioritizing time for their own self-care. For more information, please go to www.michellesegar.com.

---

* Michelle L. Segar and Caroline R. Richardson, "Prescribing Pleasure and Meaning: Cultivating Walking Motivation and Maintenance," *American Journal of Preventive Medicine* 47(6), December 2014, 838–841.

NO SWEAT

1

It's Not About the Sweat

WHEN MARCIA CALLED ME, SHE WAS AT HER WIT'S END. NOW IN HER mid-fifties, she'd been carrying around excess weight for thirty years, ever since she'd given birth to her first child. "I've tried everything," she told me, "eating special foods, fasting, diet plans from my doctor, jogging, the treadmill at the gym . . . Nothing works. I can't seem to lose weight for more than a few months at a time, and then it comes back again. I'm calling you because I know your specialty is motivation. And I need to be motivated!"

"Actually," I said, "you sound incredibly motivated. Maybe *too* motivated." I knew this would get her attention.

"How can you say I'm motivated when I'm five dress sizes bigger than I should be?" she asked. I could hear the annoyance in her voice, but I also heard the anxious pressure of *should* driving her frustration. She *should* eat less, be thinner, work out more, take care of her health

. . . Like so many of us, Marcia had come to think of food and physical movement not as the life essentials they are but as "diet" and "exercise"—a type of medicine prescribed in doses of portion sizes and reps we have to "take" or "do" to lose weight and prevent disease. But when eating and moving become something we *should* do or *have* to do rather than something we *want* to do, this undermines motivation and participation big time. After all, who looks forward to "taking her medicine"?

"Marcia," I said, "I'm going to ask you to do something, and I think it will be incredibly hard for you. But I want you to at least consider it." I didn't have to wait for her response.

"I'll do anything!" she replied, sounding ready to jump off a cliff if that's what I suggested. "Just give me a plan, a program—anything. I swear I'll follow it to a T."

"Good," I said. "I know you don't have any pressing health problems, so here's what I want you to do: I want you to stop dieting and get off that treadmill."

"And do what?" she asked.

"How about just living your life?" I responded. "How about deciding that it's okay to forget about dieting? Instead of watching calories and driving yourself to sweat, you'll begin enjoying your life by being as physically engaged in it as possible. How does that sound?"

"That *sounds* great, I guess," Marcia admitted. "But I'm not really sure what you mean by being physically engaged. And don't I have to sweat to get the benefit? Or else why do it? Honestly, I've tried just as many exercise plans as diets, and I couldn't stick with any of them. I fail with exercise, too."

"That's not a problem. I'm not going to ask you to exercise, either."

"What?!" Marcia sputtered. I think she thought I was crazy. I knew that this statement must have sounded downright insane coming from a motivation coach who specializes in getting people to become physically active.

"The idea of exercise has become too much of a synonym for punishment," I continued. "You hear the word *exercise* and immediately think that if you're not drenched in sweat and gutting it out on some kind of complicated gym equipment for at least an hour a day every day, you're failing at it."

This hit home with Marcia. "Yes! Exactly! I can't *stand* going to the gym. First, it's boring. I hate those machines and dragging myself through classes with perky instructors. Plus I'm surrounded by skinny young women who run on those treadmills as though they're outracing the bulls at Pamplona. It's so depressing!"

"So why not move your body in ways that feel good to you instead?"

The complete silence on the other end of the phone told me that Marcia had never stopped to consider this idea before. Maybe you haven't either, so let's talk about it right now.

I'm guessing that you picked up this book because, for the first or fiftieth time, you've gotten up your resolve to start exercising, watch what you eat, get in better shape, and improve your overall health. I really hope you weren't looking for another standard diet or exercise plan. Because, just as I explained to Marcia, I'm asking you to begin by doing just the opposite: Take a break. Give yourself some breathing room to consider where your usual approach to fitness and health has taken you.

The Health and Fitness Message Isn't Working

Why are so many of us on a diet and exercise treadmill, continually losing ground and gaining pounds? It's not as if we don't *want* to succeed at our fitness attempts. Each year, millions of Americans go on a diet, spending billions of dollars of their hard-earned cash on weight loss.[1] This drive for perfection is fueled by an image-obsessed culture that tells us we *need* to be more attractive and lose weight no matter what we weigh.

We hear the same health messages over and over: We're overweight. We eat too much junk. We don't exercise enough. We need to lower our blood pressure and cholesterol. We have to shed some pounds and buff up. If we don't heed this advice, we increase our risk

---

IT'S YOUR MOVE
Check Your Beliefs About What Counts

What do you believe about what makes physical movement worth doing? Please answer the following questions honestly. We'll revisit your answers later in the book.

1. In general, for exercise to "count" or be worth doing, I have to do it for _____ minutes at a time.

2. In general, I believe that for physical movement to be worth doing, I need to (circle one):

   Breathe hard and sweat

   Move

---

of cancer, diabetes, heart disease, and other illnesses. Plus, our poor health is costing us money and taxing our businesses and healthcare system. We hear these messages and others like them from our doctors, from marketers, from the news media, and even from the First Lady of the United States. And we can't argue with the underlying truth: We really *would* be better served if we got off the couch on a regular basis. We really *do* want to be healthy and fit.

So where are we going wrong? Why aren't we getting the message? As a researcher and expert on behavioral sustainability, I have spent twenty years studying these and related questions, and the truth of the matter is this: We are getting the message. We just aren't very motivated by it.

In 1994, I was working toward my first master's degree in Kinesiology, the study of human movement. (I would continue on to earn a second master's degree in Health Behavior/Health Education and a Ph.D. in Psychology.) As part of my program, my colleagues and I conducted a study to see whether ten weeks of exercise would decrease anxiety and depression among a group of breast cancer survivors.[2]

We split the participants into two groups, one that exercised and a control group that did not exercise. The results were as we expected: The survivors who exercised showed significantly lower levels of both depression and anxiety than the control group. I thought that was the end of the story until the participants came back three months later for follow-up focus groups. Not surprisingly, all of them talked about how good exercise had been for their health. But when we asked if they were still exercising, *nearly all of them said no*. When their commitment to the study ended, so did their commitment to exercise.

I was stunned—they had all reported having such good experiences with exercise. When I asked why they had stopped, they all gave the same basic reason: *We had to get back to living our lives, working, taking care of the kids and our parents* . . . Despite what they'd been through, the vast majority of the participants didn't feel compelled to continue taking care of themselves once the crisis was over. It was a shocking finding. I mean, if facing death and surviving serious illness aren't motivation enough to take better care of yourself, what is? I wanted desperately to find out.

Doing What You Enjoy Is a Better Motivator for Exercising—and It Works

Since then, I've dedicated my career to understanding the true barriers to lifelong self-care. And here's what I've found: Sensible goals or reasons for lifestyle changes—such as "preventing disease," "better health," or "weight loss"—sound great, but they exist in some vague future. We burn out long before we actually get there because the promise of a brighter day sometime down the road doesn't make us happy *right now*.

Science supports this big time. As you'll learn in this book, research shows that human beings are hardwired to choose immediate gratification over benefits we have to wait to receive. Logic doesn't motivate us—emotions do. But there is real science behind the idea that moving our bodies changes our brains in ways that lead to happiness and much more. The benefits that research shows for regular exercise are truly astounding: more energy, better sleep, less stress, less depression, enhanced mood, improved memory, less anxiety, better sex life, higher life satisfaction, more creativity, and better well-being overall.

As a scientist, educator, and motivation and self-care coach, I work with all sorts of people—some thin, some heavy, some very heavy, some healthy, some living with chronic illness. Most of my clients are women, but I've worked with men as well. And unlikely as it sounds, I've found an accessible no-cost solution that guides people to *stay* physically active, consistently take care of their bodies, have more energy, and feel better about themselves and their lives.

I've been doing research on the messages and methods of sustainable behavior change, and teaching the system on which this book is based, for almost twenty years. I've delivered the system to individual clients around the world in person, on the phone, and via Skype. I've brought it to people through hospitals and community centers, training health and wellness professionals globally. I've consulted with international corporations on their fitness apps, customer experience, and wellness programming. And I've advised healthcare companies in using my methods to improve patient behavioral sustainability, an essential element to achieve better health in people who are well or live with chronic illness.

Thanks to funding from a National Institutes of Health grant, I was able to study my program's long-term effects. The failure rate of most physical activity programs is well known: In general, most people drop out only six months after starting. By contrast, on average, ten months after my program ended, the majority of participants *sustained* an average 65 percent increase in physical activity (compared to baseline).[3] I am very passionate about my work, but it's worth noting that I have trained others to teach it, so its success rate is not just the result of my enthusiasm for it.

One key is the realization that reaping the benefits of physical activity is *not just about the sweat*: An almost infinite variety of physical movement choices and intensities will work just as well, or better, than a strict regimen of intense workouts—especially when people have chosen activities they actually enjoy doing. This statement may seem radical to you. But in fact, it is right in line with the most recent physical activity recommendations and the latest scientific findings:

» Life-centered activities such as house cleaning, gardening, and walking "count," and even just sitting less can be of benefit.

» The scientific community has given us the green light to accumulate the physical activity we do throughout our day instead of having to do it all at once.

» Our movement intensity does not have to be "vigorous" (or very hard to do) or make us sweat to "count."

As a behavioral sustainability researcher and self-care coach, I know that helping people understand these guidelines—and believe that they are true!—is crucial to helping them create physically active lifestyles that they can and want to sustain.

My coaching clients are smart people who come to me for a variety of reasons: frustration over their inability to lose weight; a gym membership that started with a firm intention to stick to a program and ended with months of paying for a membership they never use; a need to get fit because of a pressing health concern; or feeling ready to go from just trying to survive every day to genuinely thriving. They are sick and tired of short-term, one-size-fits-all solutions that preach losing weight as the key goal and never deliver results that stick. They want a new approach to self-care, well-being, health, and fitness that understands and treats them as a whole person. And, of course, they want it to work.

An Individualized Program That Changes Lives

I know it seems impossible, given the number of times you tried yet another exercise or diet plan only to watch it fall by the wayside, but my clients actually make a 180-degree turnaround in four to six weeks, and they rarely if ever change direction again. I know, because I make it a practice to follow up. When I check in with former clients years and even decades after we stopped working together, I hear the term "life-changing" over and over again. In fact, more than one of my clients has exclaimed at some point in our process of working together, "I thought this was about me learning how to get healthy and fit. But it's really about *my life*." And, I have to admit, they're right. Because face it—your health and well-being don't exist in a vacuum but in the context of your busy, crazy, complex, unpredictable day-to-day life.

My program is based on your desire to make self-care a priority and a good fit with *your* life. That's why there is nothing you "should" do; no one will stand over you to tell you "what" to do or how long or hard to do it. You don't need to buy special outfits or equipment, and you can start right where you are—in your office, your kitchen, your backyard, your neighborhood. There's only one basic instruction: Take any and every opportunity to move, in any way possible, at whatever speed you like, for any amount of time. Do what makes you feel good; stop doing what makes you feel bad. We'll talk about the details as we go along.

Your MAPS and How to Use Them

This no-strict-diet, no-do-it-till-it-burns workout attitude opens up an entirely new way to think about fitness and health that will radically transform your beliefs about what's possible, as well as your approach to your own self-care. It also requires you to start on a journey to a new way of thinking about things. That requires the right map—or, in this case, MAPS, which is how my program is structured. MAPS stands for Meaning, Awareness, Permission, and Strategy. We'll get to that in a moment.

The old maps you've tried to follow to fitness and health are very likely the ones you've been sold by the diet and exercise industry, and they likely haven't led you to physical activity that you enjoy or stay motivated to do. The MAPS I have developed will help you learn how to enjoy the benefits of daily physical movement every day, for life. MAPS is a flexible, safe, science-based approach to exercise and self-care that you can tailor to your own changing needs across a day, a week, and a lifetime.

The chapters in the first three parts of this book (Meaning, Awareness, and Permission) are the MAP that guides you on the path from where you are now to a new horizon—successfully incorporating physical movement and self-care into your life so you can feel great and fuel what matters most. You'll use the chapters in the final part (Strategy) to guide your next steps as you move forward on this new path each day, negotiating life's challenges and gifts with resilience and confidence, sustaining self-care for a lifetime.

Throughout the book—starting in this chapter—are *It's Your Move* exercises that ask you to reflect on your personal relationship with the material you're reading. Please approach these exercises in the way that works best for you. Although you may choose to write your answers directly in the book, some of the later questions call for more space than can be included here. I suggest keeping all of your responses in a separate notebook or in a special file on your laptop or tablet.

Here's a quick tour of the territory we'll cover:

> » *Meaning.* We often don't give thought to what something means to us, yet everything in our lives is symbolic and holds a personal significance that affects how we feel about it, how we approach it, and how it motivates us. The chapters in this part

will help you uncover your hidden expectations, the reasons that set you up for short-term results, and will help you understand that you can change a Meaning that leads to failure into a Meaning that motivates you to move.

» *Awareness.* What's *really* been keeping you from staying motivated? What activities fuel you, make you feel great, give you energy, and help restore you? The chapters in this part will give you Awareness of the realities of physical exercise, how you make decisions, how motivation works, and how to convert your Meaning of exercise from a chore into a gift. You'll also become aware of new science on what counts and on how easy and fun it actually is to fit and negotiate feel-good physical activities into your daily life. The *It's Your Move!* game will also help you discover the hidden opportunities to move that are hiding in plain sight. You'll learn how to gift yourself with movement in many new ways!

» *Permission.* What would your day look like if you gave yourself Permission to put self-care at the top of your to-do list? Family, work, friends, and the duties and tasks of daily life all compete for our time and energy. But self-care is not just something to do if you can find the time: Giving yourself Permission to prioritize your own self-care—to feel better every day—provides the fuel for your cherished roles and responsibilities and powers your sense of well-being.

» *Strategy.* We start with the end in mind: lifelong physical activity and well-being. We have all the best intentions in the world. Then life happens. The daily tasks, the needs of others, and our own routines present challenges that we need to meet with creative solutions. What physical activity do you want to do today? How will you accomplish it? Whom do you need to discuss it with? What will you do if something gets in your way?

The chapters in this final part get down to the nitty-gritty: evidence-based negotiation Strategies that will set you up for sustainable success and keep you there.

Your MAPS will help you redirect your thinking about physical movement and head in a new and different direction, toward satisfying and sustainable physical activity goals and outcomes, including energy, meaning, and well-being (just to name a few). In every chapter, you'll find the *It's Your Move* exercises that I use with my clients. Filling them out as you read gives you an opportunity to become more mindful of your own beliefs and experiences, to assess where you are along the path, and to uncover your core self-care needs as well as recognize what has been getting in your way of taking good care of yourself. By the end of *No Sweat*, you will have discovered many new things about yourself, what motivates you, and how you can make it all work—for life.

Influential thinkers discuss the self as a "self-system" that guides our actions to achieve the physical, emotional, and social states or well-being that we value.[4] Julius Kuhl, an internationally renowned expert on goals, motivation, and self-regulation, wrote that people's goals can't motivate self-regulation and behavior until they have *personal meaning*, through connecting with "the self."[5] Consider what "self-regulation" actually means: managing our *selves*! No wonder the "self" has to be the starting place if we aim to go beyond *changing* behavior to *sustaining* it.

This perspective helps us understand that we are dynamic beings continually striving toward what we feel and what we most cherish out of our beliefs. So if our ultimate goal is to sustain a specific self-care behavior like physical activity across our lifetime, we need to understand our beliefs about that behavior, what it symbolizes to us, and especially how it contributes to the outcomes we want from it, within the greater system of our self, our personality, and our life.

It's Your Move

You're probably wondering what happened to Marcia, the client I described at the start of this chapter. She began by deciding that she could at least pretend to think of her body as something to be taken care of and valued rather than something that needed "fixing," and to see what that would look like. This simple "let's pretend" exercise opened up a whole world of movement possibilities for Marcia. She paid attention to how much activity she was already doing—walking from her car to her office, going downstairs to the laundry room and back up again, taking walks with her dog. She stopped trying to make the treadmill work for her and began to take opportunities to move that gave her pleasure—first gardening, then riding a bike. If she didn't like something, she didn't do it again. She was surprised when, after a few weeks, she realized that she was thoroughly enjoying her new routine and felt great. And she lost some weight along the way, without even trying.

You really can make enormous changes in a relatively short time, as Marcia did, but I strongly encourage you to go at your own pace. Please do not feel pressured to achieve any benchmarks. That is the opposite of what we are doing here! If you are intrigued by what you are reading and inspired to take your self-care into your own hands, answer the following *It's Your Move* questions and consider your responses, try out the movement suggestions, relax, and have fun with it.

Here's what you *can* do: Take any and every opportunity to move, in any way possible, at whatever speed you like, for any amount of time. As previously stated, do what makes you feel good and stop doing what makes you feel bad. (We'll talk about the details as we proceed through the book.) And now that you have an overview of what's to come in *No Sweat*, let's take a look at what's most important to you through identifying your personal projects.

IT'S YOUR MOVE
Your Personal Projects List

The MAPS approach takes your entire life context into consideration—the activities, goals, tasks, and concerns that you have every day. Brian Little, a scholar in the field of personality and motivational psychology currently at Cambridge University, calls these *personal projects*.[6]

We all have a number of these personal projects that we think about, plan for, carry out, and sometimes (though not always) complete. Some personal projects may be focused on achievement (for example, learning to play the piano) or obtaining something (getting that promotion). Other personal projects focus on the process (spending time with your family, being a better parent, trying to relax more). They may be things you choose to do (read a book for pleasure), things you have to do (get your teeth cleaned, find a second job), things you are working toward (that trip to the Galapagos, learning to control your temper), or things you are trying to avoid (going into debt, fighting with your partner). They may be related to any aspect of your daily life, home, work, leisure, community—anything. Research on these ideas suggests that human flourishing is enhanced when individuals are engaged in the pursuit of personal projects that reflect who they are and what they care most about.[7]

Take a few minutes right now to think about which personal projects are most important to you in your everyday life. Now write down the *five most important personal projects* that you are currently engaged in or considering:

1. _____
2. _____
3. _____
4. _____
5. _____

Hang onto your answers. We'll revisit your list later in the book.

The Takeaways

- The health and fitness message about physical fitness isn't working to get most people to *keep* exercising.

- Doing what you enjoy is a better motivator for sustained physical activity than exercising because you think you *should* exercise.

- Your new MAPS (Meaning, Awareness, Permission, and Strategy) will help redirect your thinking about physical movement and self-care and get you headed in a new and different direction, toward personal meaning, well-being, and more satisfying goals and sustainable outcomes.

- Start by taking any and every opportunity to move, in any way possible, at whatever speed you like, for any amount of time.

PART I

• • • • •

MEANING

Your MEANING for exercise creates

your relationship with and approach to exercise.

2

Escaping the
Vicious Cycle of Failure

WHEN JACK'S DOCTOR CALLED WITH THE TEST RESULTS FROM HIS annual physical, the busy school administrator and father of two teens wasn't surprised to hear that his cholesterol was too high and his blood pressure was "borderline." His doctor had already told Jack that he could stand to lose fifteen pounds. He'd heard something similar last year as well—only then it was just ten pounds. The doctor suggested that Jack could probably control his weight with some life-style changes, and Jack resolved to finally do something about his health. He would start eating healthier to lower his cholesterol, join a gym, and begin an exercise regime.

It's a familiar tale, and for Jack it had a familiar ending. Jack started out with the best of intentions: He paid for a gym member-ship, hired a trainer, and consulted a nutritionist. For a couple of months, things went according to plan. He worked out several times a week, ate leaner meals, and cut down on snacks and treats. He was losing weight, getting fit, and feeling better.

But then life happened—all at once. Soccer season started and, during what was supposed to be Jack's workout time, he had to shuttle his daughter back and forth to practices and games. Worse, he came up against a hard deadline at work, which meant long hours, meals eaten whenever he could fit them in, and more skipped workouts. By the time the holidays rolled around, everything from his workout schedule to his healthy eating habits had gotten blown to smithereens.

Jack made a firm New Year's resolution to get back to his diet and workout plan. He renewed his gym membership, put workout days on his calendar, and bought some new athletic shoes. But in February, as he sat on the couch watching basketball, he realized he hadn't been back to the gym. He reached for a beer and some peanuts. Peanuts had a lot of protein, so that was okay, right? And beer had vitamin B-something.

Two more months passed. Then three. Jack finally got the guts to step on the scale, which confirmed his worst fears: He'd gained five more pounds. He felt like a total failure. When he thought about starting up with his diet and exercise routine again, all he felt was dread.

Then, in a casual conversation with a friend, he heard about one of my workshops. He attended one that was near his office and soon after booked a personal appointment. One of the first questions I asked him was what Meaning exercise and diet had for him. He was bewildered. "I've never thought about it," he said. "At first I want to work out, and then I just don't. Right now? Exercise just means failure and humiliation."

Does Jack's situation sound similar to yours? Have you ever joined a gym, only to have your membership go unused after the first few weeks? Have you started a diet or exercise program that you just can't sustain, even though you truly meant to make it work?

I can practically guarantee that you've been through one, if not both, of these scenarios. I know this because the vast majority of people today struggle to lead a healthy, active lifestyle only to see their good intentions and best-laid plans evaporate. (Some estimates put the percentage of unused gym memberships as high as 67 percent![1]) I call this epidemic of starting-quitting-starting-quitting the Vicious Cycle of Failure, and it's the only way most of us have learned to exercise and care for our bodies.

No one sets out to fail. Jack certainly didn't. He started out with energy and purpose. Yet Jack is almost surely going to go through the same cycle again next year, when his doctor delivers another "time to lose weight and get healthy" speech. When it comes to sticking to diet and exercise programs, failure seems to be a given. After going through this cycle a few times, people like Jack even stop going to their annual exams so they can avoid feeling a sense of failure as well as judgment from their clinicians for not having achieved their exercise or weight loss objectives.

When we decide it's time to focus on our body shape or health, we rarely stop to ask ourselves how we're thinking and feeling about this big change we want to make in our lives. Instead, we jump to the *doing* part. It happens all the time. We believe we can go from rarely exercising to becoming the image of that active and fit person we have in our minds. We expect this approach to succeed, and we feel like failures when it doesn't.

Why do we keep running up against the same wall? We already know success doesn't work that way. It's a little bit like expecting to get an A on your math test without first going to class and reading the textbook. But knowing and believing are two different things. We have a hard time ridding ourselves of the false assumption that we can achieve our fitness goals without doing the work because so much of our advertising and popular culture focuses on instant results: Just do it! Lose ten pounds overnight! Leap tall buildings in a single bound! Who doesn't want such things to happen?

It's natural to yearn for and even believe in an easy answer, a magic bullet that will finally be our salvation. But a real solution requires taking time to reflect on the societal, cultural, and familial messages that have been shaping our beliefs about physical activity for so many years. This deep understanding is the *real* magic bullet that will let us develop and take ownership of our personalized maps to long-term behavior and better results. The first step is to understand how the Meaning we hold for exercise affects our relationship with it.

What Does Exercise Mean to You?

Let's start with a basic, straightforward question: What does the word *exercise* mean to you?

Okay, so maybe that question isn't as simple as it sounds. According to cognitive scientist Benjamin K. Bergen, "Making meaning . . . [is] something we're doing almost constantly . . . What's perhaps most remarkable about it is that we hardly notice we're doing anything at all."[2] Without even realizing it, our Meaning for a behavior is constructed from what we learn about it through living in our society (the media, our culture and communities, conversations with health professionals, etc.), as well as our own personal experiences with being physically active.[3] Although you may rarely stop to consider what something means to you, everything in our lives does have a deeper symbolic Meaning that is unique to *us*. And our automatic decisions and reflexive responses to all sorts of things in our lives, including exercise, are determined by these Meanings. It is essential to understand our Meaning of physical activity because research shows that our Meanings powerfully influence our subsequent motivation, decisions, how we cope with challenges, and ultimately whether we sustain physically active lives.[4]

IT'S YOUR MOVE
Your History with Exercise

We continually get messages that influence our Meanings. Our role models, including parents, friends, and celebrities, consciously or unconsciously influence the Meanings we hold. The companies that market products to us—cars, phones, running shoes—have purposely branded them in specific ways so we develop specific messages. Take a moment now to consider what you've learned about the Meaning of being physically active and exercising from your family, friends, and the media.

1. When you were growing up, what messages (verbal or nonverbal) did you get from your family, friends, and community about exercise? (For example, who was physically active in your family? What were you told about the "right" way to exercise?)

2. What adjectives come to mind to describe the images of people exercising that you typically see in the media?

3. What do you think these images are trying to sell you?

4. How have these images made you feel about yourself? How do they make you feel about exercising?

5. What have these images motivated you to do? What do these images motivate you *not* to do?

6. Based on your answers to the questions above, what does exercise mean or symbolize to you?

The Vicious Cycle of Failure

As I said earlier, I call the cycle of try, fail, try again, fail again the Vicious Cycle of Failure. It is vicious because it sets us up to fail again and again and again—despite our best intentions. And every failure, every bad experience, reinforces the Meaning we hold for exercise. This Meaning, if you haven't guessed it already, is bound to be negative. Figure 2-1 illustrates this cycle.

FIGURE 2-1. The Vicious Cycle of Failure.

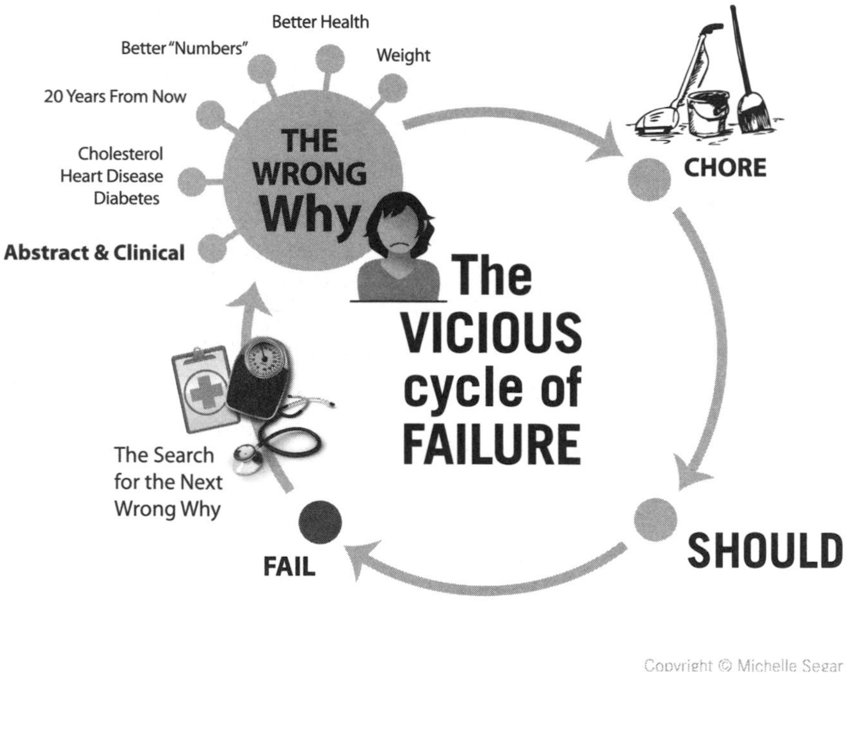
Better Health
Better "Numbers"
Weight
20 Years From Now
Cholesterol
Heart Disease
Diabetes
Abstract & Clinical
THE WRONG Why
CHORE
The VICIOUS cycle of FAILURE
The Search for the Next Wrong Why
FAIL
SHOULD
Copyright © Michelle Segar

As you can see, the Vicious Cycle of Failure always starts on the upper left side with what I call the "Wrong Why"—an initial motivation for starting a diet or exercise program that sets us up to fail before we start. You may "hate" the way you look or want to "look good" in a swimsuit, impress someone you desire, or follow your doctor's orders. Whatever the impetus for change, the Wrong Why often originates outside ourselves, to meet a societal standard or please someone.

Once we have the Wrong Why, we move into the doing it or "*chore*" phase—vowing to cut carbs, work out intensely, eat "sensibly," or whatever it takes to achieve our objective. It feels like a *should*. We do it anyway—until, inevitably, something gets in the way. We falter, we miss workouts, we eat something "bad." Eventually, we throw in the towel. *Failed* again.

After some time devoted to feeling bad about ourselves and our failure, we jump back on the cycle and start all over again—ever hopeful, but poorly motivated by *the Next Wrong Why* that sooner or later dooms us to failure again.

The obvious question is the same one I asked the study participants I told you about in Chapter 1: Why on earth do we keep doing the same thing again and again when it has led to failure?

We do it because of the Meaning we hold for exercise.

IT'S YOUR MOVE
Why Did You Start Exercising?

Take a moment to think about why you started exercising, either currently or at some time in the past. Then complete the following sentence:

Most of the time, my primary reason to begin exercising regularly has been because I have wanted to

_____.

Why We Choose the Wrong Reasons for Exercising

What physical activity means to us is the root of our motivation for doing it.[5] If our Meaning is negative, the good news is that we can change it to be positive and motivating. But we can transform our Meaning only by deconstructing it to its core parts. Our Meaning for exercise is constructed out of not only our knowledge and feeling about it from our past socialization and experiences with it but also from our *primary motivation*: in other words, the Why, the underlying reason we are choosing to do it in the first place. A negative Meaning (such as "I have to exercise hard to fix my horrible body") feels like a chore; it sets us up for negative experiences or even complete avoidance. But a positive Meaning (such as "Working out is a tool that reduces the stress I feel about my job") is a gift we want to give to ourselves. It makes us *want* to exercise.

The most common answer to the question you just answered about the primary reason to begin exercising regularly is "to lose weight." But sometimes people tell me they start exercising to become "healthier" or even to become healthier *and* lose weight. Those sound like reasonable answers, right? Well, maybe not.

As it turns out, research shows that even reasons that sound very sensible and important may not lead us to the results we're seeking. Some years ago, my colleagues and I conducted a study in which we examined the impact of people's reasons to start exercising on their actual involvement in exercise.[6] We first asked the participants to state their reasons or goals for exercising, as I just asked you. Then, to uncover their higher-level reasons for exercising, we asked them why they cared about obtaining those particular benefits. My colleagues and I found that 75 percent of participants cited weight loss or better health (current and future) as their top reasons for exercising; the other 25 percent exercised in order to enhance the quality of their daily lives (such as to create a sense of well-being or feel centered). Then we measured how much time they actually spent exercising over the course of the next year. The answer may seem counterintuitive, but it's true: The vast majority of the participants whose goals were weight loss and better health spent the *least* amount of time exercising overall—up to 32 percent less than those with other goals.

Think about that for a moment: Our most common and culturally accepted reasons for exercising are associated with doing the *least* amount of exercise. How can this be? These are sensible goals, the same goals our doctors and other health experts are always pushing. So why don't they work very well?

The answer lies in human nature. Human beings, it turns out, are hardwired to choose immediate gratification over long-term benefits. (We'll go into this science in more detail in the Awareness part of the book.) We like to think of ourselves as reasonable creatures, but logic doesn't motivate us nearly as much as our emotions do.[7] We approach what feels good and avoid what feels bad.[8] So a negative overall Meaning for exercise coupled with a payoff we have to wait years for strongly influences whether we decide to do it on a regular basis.

As motivating reasons for exercise, weight loss and better health are the Wrong Whys for many people because they do not provide the immediate rewards and feedback we need to consistently do it.[9] The results you may have been looking for will happen only down the road, *after many weeks and months* of exercise, if at all. How is that potential, far-off reward from exercising supposed to motivate you right now, today, when you need to drag yourself off the couch and get to the gym? Or when you are managing a sick kid and a looming work deadline? More often than not, it doesn't.

These types of goals are vague, gauzy images of a possible better future. There's no hard and fast promise of a better today, a shinier right now. And yet, even though these goals don't provide the immediate payoff we crave, we keep choosing them. My contention is this: *It's time to stop choosing the wrong reasons for exercising.*

Think about it. It doesn't matter whether or not things like weight loss or better health are "good" or actual goals that we or our doctors want us to achieve. It does matter, however, that they are generally *ineffective* because they don't make physical activity explicitly relevant to our most important daily roles and priorities. As a result, these types of goals don't imbue exercising with the type of Meaning that has the positivity and potency to consistently motivate most of us to be physically active for life.

It's easy to get stuck in the Vicious Cycle of Failure, but escaping this cycle is equally easy. When it comes to making a sustainable change in your behavior, understanding your *Meaning* is your starting place because it determines the tone of your relationship with being physically active (or any behavior). In practical terms, your Meaning for being physically active determines whether or not you will make time, day after day, to do it and ultimately whether you achieve your desired goals from physical activity.

IT'S YOUR MOVE
Are You Starting from the Wrong Why?

Go back and look at your response to the *It's Your Move* question "Why did you start exercising?" earlier in this chapter. If you start out by choosing the wrong reasons for beginning to exercise, you're ensuring failure before you even get going.

Based on what you wrote, do you think you've been starting from the Wrong Why?

Escaping Your Personal Vicious Cycle of Failure

Every failure at sticking to a workout program, and every bad experience you have with exercise, reinforces the way you view exercise and keeps you at war with your body:

» You maintain a *negative* Meaning for exercise.

» You set *unachievable* weight- or body-related exercise goals.

» You feel *discouraged* about your ability to be physically active.

» You come to *dislike* being physically active.

Does reading this list motivate you to be physically active? Of course it doesn't. For most of us, exercise is a means to an end sometime in the future. We do it because we want to look better or be healthier or fit back into that pair of tiny jeans we bought years ago. We do it because we are out to achieve some long-term health-related goal like decreasing our risk of heart disease or lowering our cholesterol. So please set those reasons aside for now, at least until you've finished reading this book.

You may think I'm crazy. Here I am, a professional in the health field, and I'm asking you for now to forget about health factors as your motivator. But I don't ask lightly. I ask because I don't want you to fail now, or fail again. If you fail, it doesn't matter how good your intentions were when you started. Right now, let's really pin down your personal Meaning for exercise: When you think about exercise, does it feel like a chore you *have* to do? Or like a gift you can't wait to open?

IT'S YOUR MOVE
A Chore or a Gift?

On a scale of 1 to 5—with 1 being "a chore to accomplish" and 5 being "a gift to give yourself"—circle the number that best describes how you feel about exercise:

1   2   3   4   5

Chore   Gift

If your answer to the above question landed closer to the "gift" end of the spectrum, you're ahead of the game. The ideas and approaches you'll learn in the rest of this book will add to your enjoyment and show you new ways to ensure that this is a gift you will continue to open for a lifetime.

But if you said that physical activity feels like a chore, then it's something you're doing because you feel like you *should*, not because you want to. When something feels like a chore, we tend to put off doing it and find any reason to avoid it. It's going to be pretty hard, if not impossible, to make a chore a sustainable part of your life.

But please, don't give up now. Instead, consider this: *Physical activity doesn't have to feel like a chore.* We'll dive into this startling idea in the next chapter. But before we do, you probably have a question.

Do You Just Need More Willpower?

At this point in the conversation (or even earlier!), this is what I often hear: "That's all very interesting about meaning and motivation, Michelle, but it won't help me. I just have to muster up more willpower."

Well, guess what? When your exercise depends on your having "enough" willpower or self-control to consistently power through both your ambivalence and your feeling that exercise is a chore, you've chosen a strategy that fails most people. Two studies show the very real limitations of willpower, which is also called "ego depletion."

Researchers in one classic study used two groups of dieters to observe the effects of using willpower, or self-control, to resist sweets while watching a video.[10] One group had close access to an overflowing bowl of candy, while the other group was asked to sit far away from the candy. In addition, some participants were told they could go ahead and eat the candy, while others were asked not to eat the candy because it was needed for another study later that day. The experiment was structured to tempt some of the dieters with the candy so they would have to use willpower to resist temptation, while the other participants did not have to exert self-control at all. But what these investigators were really interested in was how these different groups would respond in the second part of the experiment.

Following the video, both groups were allowed to have as much ice cream as they wanted in the guise of "rating" flavors. The investigators then measured how much each participant ate. Their hypothesis turned out to be correct: The dieters who had been placed close to the candy in the first part of the study and were told it was okay to eat it—thus needing to exert their self-control (they were dieters, remember)—ate significantly more ice cream compared to the dieters who sat far from the candy or were instructed not to eat it, and thus did not need to exert self-control.

This study shows that *using self-control or willpower in one situation can deplete it in a future situation.* It's like sand running through an hourglass. We have a finite amount of self-control—and the more we use it, the less we have. In fact, using functional neuroimaging, or fMRI (technology that measures areas and relationships in the brain), scientists can now actually watch the mechanisms that underlie the depletion of willpower in the brain.

A second study, done with a group of thirty-one chronic dieters (individuals who tried diet after diet to lose weight), examined changes in the participants' brain activity in response to viewing desirable foods.[11] Before viewing the foods, half of the dieters completed a task known to deplete willpower. Compared with the dieters who did not do this task, the dieters whose willpower had been depleted exhibited a greater response to food cues in reward centers of the brain (the orbitofrontal cortex), along with decreased ability to communicate to another part of the brain implicated in self-control (the frontal gyrus). In this case, seeing is believing: Using self-control in a prior situation actually influences our brain and impacts the potential to use it later.

These findings suggest that just participating in a depleting task results in future self-control failure! Think about it. How many depleting tasks do you already perform in one day (taking care of children, doing your job, studying for exams, taking care of your parents)? The normal stress of life may actually reduce the way your brain responds to self-control, further decreasing its capacity to resist temptation.

So please: Forget about willpower as the chief approach for achieving lasting behavior change. It's not that you can't build up your willpower because, to some extent, you can. But even though we can increase our willpower capacity through valuable activities like getting more sleep[12] and even practicing self-control,[13] that doesn't mean that we should consider it as our primary plan for sustainability. The fact remains that willpower depletes with use. Depending on a resource that is known to deplete with use? Not a good idea for the long run. But there is a much more dependable and stable system that reflects who you are and what is most meaningful to you. Because it reflects who you are instead of depleting you, this system actually energizes you when you use it, generating a positive and renewable source of motivation that has the potency to fuel lasting results. In the next chapter, we'll start to explore this self-system that resides *inside you* and how it holds the key to converting your Meaning of exercise from a chore into a gift.

The Takeaways

- Research shows that people's most common motivations for exercising—weight loss and better health—have actually been associated with doing the least amount of exercise.

- The Vicious Cycle of Failure begins with the Wrong Why—an externally motivated (*should*), abstract, or future-oriented reason for starting a new behavior like exercise.

- The Vicious Cycle of Failure sets you up to fail at exercise and diet programs over and over again, regardless of your best intentions, reinforcing the negative Meaning you hold for exercise and making you feel bad about yourself. But escaping the Vicious Cycle of Failure is easier than you think.

- Meaning is the root of your motivation. A negative, chore-based Meaning for exercise leads to poor motivation; a positive, gift-like Meaning for exercise leads to high-quality motivation.

- You acquire your Meaning for exercise unconsciously, through your socialization (the messages of society, family, friends, and the media) and your past experiences with it.

- Your Meaning of physical activity is determined by the primary reason you initiate it (the Why) and the past experiences you've had being physically active.

- If you want to change your relationship with being physically active, the starting place is understanding and changing your Meaning of it.

- Willpower depletes with use, so it is not the most strategic system to rely on to sustain the behavioral changes that you desire.

3

Motivation from the Inside Out

TANYA, RECENTLY MARRIED AND IN HER LATE THIRTIES, CAME TO ME with a familiar problem. She had gained some weight after her marriage (weight she'd dropped for the wedding) and wanted to "get in shape." But despite a number of attempts, she couldn't seem to stick with an exercise program. She told me it was a lifelong issue.

We'd just started to talk about her Meaning for exercise, and she'd jumped on the idea of chore. "That's it *exactly*," she agreed. Then she abruptly changed the subject and began complaining about how much it irritated her when her husband went running—especially when he left the house looking positively gleeful about what he was about to do. "He *loves* it," she said, shaking her head in disgust. "He'll even give up other things I know he enjoys, like watching baseball games or meeting his friends, just so he can get in his run. He ran track in school and everything. Exercise is such a natural thing for him. It's *so* annoying. I really don't get it."

"Let me make sure I understand what you're saying," I said. "You resent your husband because he *wants* to go running, while you feel like exercising is something you *have* to do."

"Yes," she replied, sounding almost guilty.

"You see exercise as something you don't want to do, or even as your punishment for gaining the weight. Your husband is like a kid with a birthday gift—he can't wait to open it, right?"

"I guess so," she said. "Yeah, I never thought about it that way."

"But what if you could feel gleeful about physical activity too?" I asked.

She didn't say anything for a moment, and I let the silence hang there so she could think about the question. It was clearly an idea that hadn't occurred to her before.

"That would be . . . amazing," she said hesitantly, "but I don't see how it's possible. I'm not a runner. I'm not built that way."

"Running may not be your thing," I said, "but the gleeful part is definitely possible. Let's take it one step at a time. You've already taken the first step—acknowledging that exercise feels like a negative to you, like a chore. That feeling reflects the Meaning being physically active has for you right now. Believe it or not, we can change that pretty easily."

"I trust you, Michelle, but I don't really believe that's true. I've felt this way for the last sixteen years, since college."

"I know that, Tanya, but once we start to better understand why you feel the way you do, you'll be surprised how effortless and quick this conversion can be."

I explained to Tanya that everything we've learned about exercise and physical activity through culture, the media, and our past experiences—I'm not good at this, it's supposed to be fun, I'm being forced to do it, it hurts, it's humiliating, it will fix my unattractive body—creates our Meaning of exercise and physical activity. "You know from your own life that thinking of exercise as a chore undermines your motivation before you even start," I said. She nodded, and I continued. "It might help for you to understand how it got to be this way for you."

Our Past Experience with Exercise Builds Our Meanings

We develop our perceptions and understanding about things over our entire lifetime, based on our own idea of how the world works that we've constructed from specific experiences and interactions,[1] especially emotional ones.[2] Whatever Meaning you ascribe to exercise, for example, is completely unique to you because it has been constructed *from your interactions* with physical activity.

We form ideas and values about all sorts of things throughout life from our experiences. It's how we try to make sense of the world. Out of these experiences we develop associations that we generalize and project into the future. For example, consider what "getting a shot" can mean to us. On the surface, it's just an objective, neutral activity, like exercising. But below the surface, "getting a shot" is embedded with our past knowledge, experiences, and emotions, such as sickness, anxiety, and pain.[3] Depending on how negative our experiences have been, just thinking about getting a shot can flood our minds and bodies with strong feelings, like dread or aversion. Even stepping into the doctor's office can activate and arouse these negative feelings because we associate the office with the shot experience. And if we had a choice, we would avoid getting a shot altogether.

In the same way, we've developed Meanings for exercise and physical activity that similarly influence us. Because these Meanings have been built through experience and knowledge, we can change them only by learning new things about exercise and physical activity and having new experiences with being physically active and exercising.

While this is plain common sense, research shows that our past experiences with any behavior strongly influence our perceptions of it, our beliefs about it, our Meaning for it, and ultimately whether we choose to do it or not.[4] I'll break this idea down because this is one of the most important points of this whole book and the secret ingredient in my MAPS method:

» Our past experiences with exercise, our past reasons for doing it, and what we have learned to believe about it (as children and as adults) combine together to generate our Meaning for exercising and being physically active.

» Our Meanings influence our perceptions and feelings about exercising *outside of our Awareness.*

» Because we tend to approach what feels good and avoid what feels bad (unconsciously, outside of our Awareness), our Meaning about physical activity powerfully influences our behavior without our even knowing it.

Many people feel ambivalent about being physically active because of their accumulation of experiences over their lifetime about why they should do it and how it feels. These are often a mix of good and bad: not being chosen for a team, being chided about being overweight by a clinician who prescribed exercise as the remedy, enjoying swimming with friends at camp, being teased in gym class, a spring hike with friends, feeling self-conscious in the gym. All of these diverse experiences form the general Meaning that physical activity has for you—*and that forms the basis of your relationship with exercise and physical activity.* In general, if your exercise history has been predominantly or especially negative, the Meaning it has for you now also feels negative: It's a chore. If exercise has been positive for you over time and you've chosen to do it because *you* wanted to, then physical activity is likely to have a positive Meaning for you: It's a gift you want to give to yourself. Even with early positive experiences and a positive Meaning about sports or physical activity, later negative experiences can affect your Meaning. And because our Meaning of physical activity has been constructed outside of our Awareness, we might not even realize that it exists.

Let's go back to my talk with Tanya. "Tanya," I said, "the place I always start with my clients is to help them understand their Meaning of exercise and physical activity through exploring their past experiences and reasons for starting."

She said:

Well, as a kid, I remember running around a lot with my friends and having fun with my family. But college was pretty stressful, and there was a machine in the dorm that sold chips and candy. I gained the "freshman fifteen" fast—more like twenty-five pounds in my case. I hated the way I looked in clothes. I didn't want to have anything to do with all those girls in my dorm who were going for runs in their tiny shorts. I was too embarrassed. When I was a junior, my roommate kept getting on me for just sitting on the couch, and she pushed me to sign up for these free aerobics classes they were offering on campus. I went, but I hated them. Exercise felt like a necessary evil that I just had to do to lose weight. Ever since then, I haven't been able to stick with any kind of regular exercise, although believe me, I've paid money for more than one gym membership. I feel tired every day, plus I don't want anyone to see me jumping around. All those mirrors. It's humiliating.

"It sounds like you started out with very positive Meanings for exercise, right?" I asked. Tanya nodded, listening attentively. "But as a young adult, your feelings that exercise was basically a necessary evil for weight loss crowded out that positivity. And then your Meaning became progressively *more* negative every time you forced yourself to sign up at the gym. It's a downward spiral."

"That sums it up nicely," said Tanya, starting to laugh despite the doom and gloom of her story. "I do feel like I'm just spiraling down the drain sometimes. So what's the good news?"

"Tanya, I am delighted to tell you that your situation is not unique, and it's not irreversible. Early on, your relationship with physical movement was converted from fun that you autonomously *chose* to do into a vehicle for losing weight, something you feel you *should* do that you *forced yourself* to do."

Tanya sat up straight, clearly startled. "Oh! I get it! It's like when your mom says 'Eat your vegetables, they're good for you. And you can't leave the table until you finish all of them.' So then of course you don't want to touch the veggies, ever. Right? You want to eat snacks before dinner just to prove you can make your own choices."

"Exactly," I agreed. "You've got it. And there's some good science behind what you intuitively figured out."

Self-Determination Theory Supports the Benefits of Owning Our Choices

Would you rather do something because someone in authority tells you that you *have to do it or else*? Or because you're enthusiastic and curious about the idea and motivated to try it out?

You probably don't even have to think about your answer: You'd rather be in charge of your own life decisions. Well, there's solid science behind why you feel that way, and you can use it to foster your desire and motivation for being physically active. Self-determination theory (SDT) distinguishes between feeling either "controlled" or "autonomous" toward a behavior, and it shows how these differences can affect subsequent motivation and adherence.[5] According to SDT, an individual who feels controlled toward being physically active—say, being told that she *must* take a brisk forty-minute walk every day—would consider walking a *should*. To this person, walking is something she has to do in order to avoid a punishment (such as having to pay higher healthcare premiums), to comply with an external pressure (such as following a doctor's prescription to lose weight), or just because she thinks it's "the right way" to exercise. In contrast, an individual who feels autonomous toward walking decides to do it because she *wants* to do it in the ways that she chooses to do it. This person deeply values her reasons for taking a walk, understands and acts on the benefits she gets from walking, or simply experiences pleasure or feels satisfaction from the process of being physically active.

When we experience autonomy, we feel ownership over our movement and choose activities that are meaningful and feel good to *us*. We do them on a regular basis, and we keep it up over the long term. A systematic review of SDT and physical activity and exercise found consistent support for a positive relationship between more autonomous forms of motivation and physical activity.[6] It also found that controlled forms of motivation don't work as consistently well as autonomous motivation. These findings make sense: When we feel that *who we are* is driving our decision to start taking regular walks, for example, we have higher-quality motivation—we even feel energized from doing it. We are more likely to keep up the walks, if they reflect our core needs and desires, than we are to go on walks just to comply with the nagging feeling that we *should* walk, "for our own good."

Weigh these factors: How many times have you started to exercise because you felt pressured to lose weight or to exercise in "the right way," and how often have you stuck with it? If you are reading this book, your answer is probably "every time." That's likely because the messages that have been directing your exercise choices are pressuring you instead of fueling you.

Take Ownership of Your Exercise

"Why does this keep happening? It's déjà vu all over again!"

Our old Meanings are embedded and automatic, and they keep putting us in the same familiar but uncomfortable situations: Here we are. Again. These old Meanings belong to us, but they are invisible to us because they were constructed unconsciously through our experiences. Although it often feels as if outside forces must be controlling us, we can take control at any time, changing a chore into a gift and thus altering the whole game.

A new client of mine, Charles, is an accounts manager in his early fifties. Right away, during our first phone session, he told me about how much he resented his personal trainer for pushing him so hard. "He's like a drill instructor," said Charles. "I never want to do what he tells me. It reminds me of being back in the Army."

"But wait," I said, "didn't you tell me that you hired him *because* you knew his regimen would be tough work?"

"Yes," he admitted, "I told him to push me hard. But it's torture! Sometimes I hope he'll cancel. And most times after a session I just have to lie down and tell my family to leave me alone. The next day I can barely move. I don't even want to have sex with my wife."

"It sounds pretty awful," I said. "I can see why you're fighting it. But let's look at it another way. Instead of blaming him, let's go back to why you hired him. Strange as it sounds now, you actually hired him to do just what he's doing." The silence was so thick I thought Charles might have quietly hung up. But he was just taking in what I had said.

"Yeah," he said finally, "that's true. I guess I did hire him to push me hard. And why not? I mean, I can't get myself motivated to work out hard enough on my own to make exercise worthwhile. Look, just tell me what I need to know so I can stay motivated to stick with this. My wife and doctor have both been nagging me to take better care of myself."

Charles seemed reticent to take responsibility for being the origin of the intense workout he resented doing, but he didn't deny that he had hired his trainer precisely to force him to do a tough workout regimen. He was convinced that's how you had to do it.

"I've worked out hard for six weeks now," he said. "I'm committed to it, but I hate doing it. It's exhausting and I dread it. I hired a trainer to push me so I'd lose weight, and I did lose a little, but all the effort I'm putting in is not really getting me the results I need. I don't want to just drop out and stop exercising, because I'm tired of failing every time I try this damned exercise thing."

"Wait a second," I said. "Let's bring it down to specifics. Can you tell me the part of your workout that is the worst for you?"

"That's easy. I do a four-mile run that sucks. My trainer tells me to sprint up this hill that's at about mile three, but it's a killer. I dread every session."

"You really need to stop butting heads with exercise," I said. Then I introduced the idea that physical activity can actually be a gift instead of such a chore. Charles snorted.

"To make that transformation," I continued, "you're going to need to take charge of your exercise and decide how you want to do it. Make it a gift to yourself."

"I don't want to wimp out. Plus I have no clue what you're talking about."

"Simple," I said. "Instead of *making* yourself sprint up that hill at mile three because you're *supposed* to, how about taking charge of how you move and figure out what *you* want to do and how you want to do it? Maybe you could decide to run more slowly or even *walk* up the hill instead."

"But that's cheating."

"Just try it once and see how it goes, okay? You'll still be at the top of the hill."

"I don't know," said Charles. "I don't want to give up my routine. Then I'll be back where I started. I'm prediabetic now, whatever that means."

"Look, Charles, if you are being physically active to comply with some external pressure, maybe even doing it harder than you want because you think you should, you won't do it for very long. That's not just you; it's me, and most everybody else. This is not about being tough enough to handle what your trainer is telling you to do. This is about human nature. People avoid what feels bad and strive toward what feels good."

"Uh-huh."

"If you keep exercising in ways that don't reflect you and your preferences," I continued, "eventually your motivation will peter out and you'll stop. Then you'll miss out on the incredible benefits exercise really has to offer, and your health situation will not likely improve. Plus, research clearly shows that keeping up with exercise is a critical behavior for maintaining weight loss. So sticking with exercise is fundamental to what you, your wife, and your doctor are after. I'm just asking you to think about it in a different way. Believe me, Charles, there's research showing that this program I'm suggesting really works."

At our next session, Charles called and told me something that I hadn't anticipated. I had fully expected him to say that he had stopped running up the hill altogether. Instead, he told me that as he was getting close to the hill and thinking about what he wanted to do, he had a realization: *Sprinting* up the hill was a gift that he *wanted* to give himself. I was completely surprised by his choice but really pleased. A week later, at our next session, he told me that he found himself enjoying this personal challenge of pushing himself even harder and that he was sprinting even more on the run. Exerting himself in this way now felt more like a privilege than a chore. And he no longer felt exhausted when he got home.

Talk about a quick yet transformative turnaround! By simply reframing this intense physical workout as *his choice* instead of a mandate he had to comply with, his sprint became energizing rather than depleting. And it also became a practice he happily kept up. Stories like this never cease to fascinate me, even though I've seen time and again the powerful downstream effects on our experience, our energy levels, and much more just from how we frame what we do.

Framing Is Everything: The "Work or Fun" Study

In a study aptly titled "Work or Fun?" researchers were interested in discovering whether framing an activity explicitly as either one or the other would influence people and their self-control.[7] In essence, they wanted to find out if having the same activity *mean* different things would influence outcomes.

In a series of experiments, they investigated a handful of issues related to studying the impact of framing the same activity as either work or fun. Although their findings showed that things like individual differences can also influence the outcomes, in general, they found that framing a behavior as work (an obligation) made the experience of engaging in the behavior depleting and caused participants to have more difficulty exerting self-control and finishing the task. In contrast, when the same behavior was framed as an opportunity to have fun, completing the behavior was vitalizing and made subsequent self-control easier.

This study has important implications about how we frame the reason for doing exercise and other health-related activities. If the underlying reason for the behavior feels like something we *should* do (i.e., the Wrong Why), it leads to a chore-based Meaning, and as a result, it is more likely to make performing the behavior depleting and increases the chance that we will not have the desire or energy to stick with it. We are more likely to sustain behavior like physical activity when we view it as a gift, something that is fun or personally meaningful. Supporting self-determination theory, this research suggests that our experience from doing any behavior is drastically influenced by the frame—the primary reason for doing it, our Why. The Why, in fact, is the foundation of the entire behavioral process.

The Why: The Foundation of Sustainable Behavior Change

The Why we have for adopting a new behavior reflects the end result we hope to achieve (our goal) from changing our behavior. It is more important than you may think.

Research shows that goals energize and direct behavior and are actually the *starting point* of a behavior change process.[8] In essence, the specific and primary goals we have for any behavior create the frame through which that behavior is perceived and viewed.[9] So a behavior like physical activity can be understood *only* by identifying the specific goals it aims to achieve.[10] A sub-theory of self-determination theory called goal contents theory suggests that your Why, or the outcome you hope for in making a behavior change like becoming more physically active, will determine whether you develop a more autonomous or controlling type of motivation.[11] Given that autonomous motivation is much more likely to energize you and fuel long-term behavior change than controlled motivation, it's crucial to understand which Whys lead to autonomous motivation.

In another of my studies, my colleagues and I investigated the relationships between distinct Whys for exercising and autonomous and controlling forms of motivation.[12] We found that people who exercised with health-related or weight-loss Whys reported on average 30 percent less autonomous motivation and 15 percent more controlling motivation than those participants whose Whys aimed to reduce their daily stress or enhance their well-being.

Our Why, our primary reason for initiating any behavior, influences the subsequent quality of the motivation that we develop. Consider the Why as the *source* of your fuel. Would you rather fill your car's tank with optimal, high-quality fuel that will get you to your ultimate destination? Or with off-brand, low-quality fuel that will take you a few miles and then cause your engine to sputter and conk out before you get where you're going? Clearly, the first choice is the strategic choice, the Right Why.

The Right Whys motivate us because they are relevant to our daily lives and personally meaningful. Compared to the Wrong Whys, which leave us feeling depleted, the Right Whys energize and empower us. When we choose the Right Whys for physical activity, we create our own renewable high-quality fuel *inside of ourselves*. In Chapter 6, we'll talk at length about how to discover your Right Whys. For now, I want to tell you about some fascinating new research showing that different Whys for walking also influence our energy levels and how much we eat afterward.

How Our Whys Influence Even How Much We Eat

Do you think that people experience walking differently and eat more afterward depending on their reason for walking? Researchers tackled this question head on in a couple of studies.[13]

The first study was conducted with mostly overweight but otherwise healthy women. All of the participants were provided with maps of the same one-mile outdoor course and were told that they would get lunch after their thirty-minute walk was over. Half of the women were told that their reason for walking (their Why) was to "exercise." They were encouraged to view it as such and to notice how they felt throughout the walk. The other group was told that they were walking in order to have fun. They were given music to listen to and told to enjoy themselves on the walk.

Afterward, the researchers asked each woman to calculate her mileage and calorie expenditure and to describe her mood. Both groups reported extremely similar mileage and calories burned, but they experienced the walk quite differently. The women who had been walking to exercise said they felt more tired and grumpy than the women who were exercising for fun.

Even more interesting is what happened when the women sat down to a pasta lunch. They could choose between either water or a sugary soda to drink, and between applesauce or chocolate pudding for dessert. The women who had been told that their Why for walking was to exercise took in significantly more calories from soda and pudding than the women whose Why for walking was to have fun.

The researchers conducted a follow-up experiment with both men and women that supported and added to these findings. In this second study, a different set of volunteers were asked to walk one mile. Once again, half of the participants were told that they were walking for exercise, while the others were told that their reason for walking was to take in the view and just have fun. In this second experiment, the researchers did not ask the "fun" group to listen to music as they had done in the first study because they wanted to make sure that it was the fun framing, rather than the music, that influenced the results. This study used candy instead of lunch to measure how much participants consumed. Afterward, in the guise of a thank you, all the participants were given a plastic bag and told they could fill it with as many M&Ms as they wanted. As you've probably already surmised, the volunteers from the exercise group poured in twice as many M&Ms as the volunteers who were walking for fun.

These two experiments underscore that how we frame physical activity affects how we feel about it, how depleted we feel, and the ensuing choices we make. The same exertion, spun with a Why for "fun," prompts happier moods and less gorging on high-calorie foods than a Why for "exercise."

Our Why is foundational. It has a domino effect on everything that follows: how we feel, how we behave, and our subsequent motivation to make choices that favor self-care and health.

Muddying the Waters: More Motives Are *Not* More Motivating

At this point in the conversation, clients often tell me, "Okay, Michelle, I get it, you sold me. I want to have the Right Why. I understand that it's much more motivational. But I still want to lose weight! Why can't I use physical activity to feel better and also use it for weight loss? Then I'll have *two* reasons to exercise instead of one. Won't that give me more motivation?"

Not really. In fact, research suggests the exact opposite may be true.

Exercising as a way to help you achieve something specific outside of yourself, like losing ten pounds or lowering your cholesterol by fifty points, is an *external* reason (or extrinsic goal). External reasons are sometimes called *instrumental* because they are a means to an end. In contrast, exercising because you genuinely want to, because you've chosen an activity you enjoy and are looking forward to, is an *internal* reason (or intrinsic goal) that fuels your core needs and wants: who you are.

When you put these two different motivations together, something strange happens: Multiple motives seem to decrease motivation, not enhance it. I've seen this effect in my own research and also noticed it in my work with clients over the years. The ones who try to have a few different kinds of Whys for exercise seem to be distracted by the competing outcomes they're striving to achieve: Are they exercising for weight loss? To feel better? To get healthy? As they lose focus, motivation goes out the window.

I've been fascinated to read the research that supports my observations. Amy Wrzesniewski of Yale University led a study on more than 10,000 cadets at the U.S. Military Academy at West Point to evaluate their professional success over a decade from the impact of having different types of motives for enlisting.[14] Would holding *both* internal motives (military service is personally meaningful to them) and external motives (prestige, career advancement) for joining the Army be valuable career-wise, or would such motives compete over time? The long time frame allowed Wrzesniewski and her colleagues to identify which cadets became commissioned officers, which extended their officer service beyond the minimum required period, and which were selected for early career promotions.

In each case, they found that having a personally meaningful reason for being in the service predicted the most positive outcomes. But they also found that when the cadets *also held* external reasons for enlisting, this positive relationship was undermined. These findings support the idea that having both external and internal Whys can undermine persistence and performance over long periods of time.

A very different study, on nutrition and kids, reported a very similar phenomenon.[15] In this case, researchers offered children the same food but gave different children one of three different messages along with the food: (1) It's yummy (internal); (2) it will make you strong (instrumental, external); or (3) it is yummy *and* will make you strong (internal *and* external). They hypothesized that when you make something that is intrinsically pleasant (like a cracker) into something that is also instrumental in some way (a cracker that is also good for you), it will undermine the positive effects from internal, pleasurable benefits. And that is exactly what happened. Kids who were told it was "yummy" and will make you "strong" rated the cracker as less tasty, and they ate less of it, than kids who were told only that it was yummy.

Having more than one primary Why for doing a behavior is thought to "dilute" our motivation.[16] We become less motivated and perceive a specific behavior as less effective in achieving any one goal (or Why) when it aims to achieve *more* than one. Plus, if we hold two or three different Whys for exercising and feel differently about each of them, it also generates ambivalence. And that's not good for motivation, either.[17]

Marketers understand this perfectly. Consider how the most popular companies market their products to us. They don't give us three different reasons to buy their product; they brand it with one primary meaning. They know that to really get us hooked and coming back for more, again and again, they need to identify a very strategic, emotionally focused benefit from using their product or service that we'll focus on and desire to keep having. One make of car, for example, may be "sexy," while another one is "sporty." We want one or the other but probably not both. Clearly, marketers are onto something that we can all learn from.

IT'S YOUR MOVE
More Than One Reason?

Go back to your reasons for exercise in the *It's Your Move* exercise in Chapter 2 called "Why Did You Start Exercising?" Do you currently hold more than one Why for wanting to include exercise in your life?

In this chapter we learned how central the Why is to our motivation, mood, and even other health-related decisions like eating. In the next chapter, we are going to look at the manner in which our Whys also dictate the specific physical activities we choose and the reasons these choices are critical for our ultimate success.

The Takeaways

* You develop your Meanings for things over your entire lifetime. You are often not explicitly aware of the Meaning behavior has for you.

* You can change your Meaning of a behavior only by having new experiences and learning new things that will enable you to construct a new Meaning. Changing your Meaning for exercise can help you take ownership of it and feel more in control of your physical activity choices.

* Self-determination theory holds that when you experience ownership over what you are doing (autonomy), you choose activities that are meaningful and feel good to *you*, you are more likely to do them on a regular basis, and you keep them up over the long term, compared to doing them because you think you *should*.

* How a behavior is framed by the primary reason for doing it impacts how that behavior affects you, including your energy level, your self-control, and even how much you eat.

* The Why is the foundation of the entire behavior change process. The Why you have for adopting a new behavior—your reason for doing it—reflects the end result you hope to achieve from changing your behavior.

* The Right Whys are the motivators of sustainable behavior change

because they reflect roles and goals and are very personally compelling. They are energizing and empowering.

- Having multiple motivations (both Wrong Whys and Right Whys) for doing a behavior is actually *less motivating*. They compete with each other, dilute your motivation, and create ambivalence, undermining your desire to stick with physical activity.

PART II

• • • • •

AWARENESS

AWARENESS helps you identify what's been standing

in your way and discover physical activities

that motivate you.

4

Exorcising Exercise

SANDY TOLD ME THAT SHE HAD BEEN STRUGGLING WITH HER WEIGHT all of her adult life. She wasn't overweight all the time; it was more that her weight seesawed—sometimes up, sometimes down, then up again, then back down. As she explained it to me, "When I feel like I've gained too much weight, I drag myself to the gym to do the elliptical and other machines for a few weeks. I get my weight down, but then I get bored and stop going. And I start gaining weight again."

When I asked her why she keeps going back to the gym if she has to drag herself there and it bores her, she replied, "What else would I do? I know that's what I should be doing."

"Isn't there some other activity you could try?" I asked.

"Well, I really like walking outside . . ."

"Then why not do that?"

"Because it doesn't feel like it counts as exercise."

"Why?"

Sandy didn't really have an answer for that, just vague notions that some types of exercise "counted" while others didn't, and the ones that counted were what she *should* be doing.

Nearly all the clients I've worked with over the years have told me that they've forced themselves to do various kinds of exercise that they don't really like doing. But when I ask them why they choose activities they don't like instead of something they do like, they really don't know. But I do: It's because they are starting from the Wrong Why.

Sandy's Wrong Why was "to lose weight." This guided her to choose intense physical activities at the gym that she thought she *should* do in order to burn calories. But although this tactic helped her meet her goal in the short term, it didn't work for her in the long run. Because she didn't like working out at the gym, she didn't stay motivated or have the energy to keep making herself go once her short-term goal was accomplished. She had set herself up for the Vicious Cycle of Failure, and she came to accept that it was the only way.

Body-Shaping and Weight-Loss Whys Guide Us to Work Out in Ways We Don't Like

My colleagues and I conducted a study to see if a focus on weight and body shape affected the way midlife women of similar age and weight approached being physically active.[1] We identified two groups based on what the women wrote in answer to this prompt: "Imagine that you are being physically active right now. Take a minute or two and go over the experience in your mind." Then we asked them to describe what they were feeling and thinking in three or four sentences. Participants who wrote down terms like "calories," "weight," or "how I look" were put into a group we called "body-shapers." Those who didn't write any terms related to body weight and shape we called "non-body-shapers."

We noticed right away that body-shapers and non-body-shapers wrote very differently about being physically active. For example:

» *Body-shaper:* "I'm feeling winded and uncomfortable. I do feel better for making an effort to get into shape. Hoping that I can keep it up!"

» *Non-body-shaper:* "Feels good to be moving. Feels good to be outside."

The difference in tone between the two groups was apparent. The non-body-shapers mentioned getting pleasure from moving their bodies more often, while the body-shapers expressed more struggle, particularly with the need to lose weight. (Remember: On average, both groups weighed the same.) The body-shapers also used the expression "I should" more than the non-body-shapers, reflecting a controlling type of motivation that is not optimal for long-term change. In contrast, the non-body-shapers expressed more intrinsic motivation and wrote more about feeling good and enjoying being physically active.

We wanted to know whether these groups of women did differing amounts of exercise. They did: The women with body-shaping motives exercised almost 40 percent *less* than those who were not exercising to shape their bodies.

Then we wondered why the body-shapers were not as motivated to exercise. Were they choosing different types of physical activities than non-body-shapers? Indeed, they were. The body-shapers reported participating in structured or formal exercises, such as aerobic exercise classes, *three times more* than the non-body-shapers. In addition, only 15 percent of the body-shapers reported walking compared to more than 50 percent of the non-body-shapers! And there was another interesting finding: The women who were exercising to get their bodies into shape reported more negative feelings *about being physically active* than the women who were exercising for non-body-shape reasons.

This study was an eye-opener. When we choose to move in ways that don't feel good, most of us are likely—I'd say predictably—*not* going to keep it up. Exercising to lose weight puts us on a path that leads straight to picking exercises that we do not like just so we can burn the most calories as quickly as possible. Sure, these punishing exercises might burn more calories in the two weeks that we do them. But how many calories will we ultimately burn from these exercises if we can't motivate ourselves to get to the gym on a regular basis?

And therein lies the problem: Choosing to move in ways that feel punishing so you can burn the most calories is very strategic if you have a short-term goal. But if your goal is to maintain physical activity over a lifetime and reap the multitude of benefits it brings, try to refocus and start choosing to move in ways that feel good to you. That's because the best determinant of sustainability is not how much weight you hope to lose but *how participating in physical activities makes you feel* in the moment.

To Feel or Not to Feel?: Feelings Trump Function

According to current thinking, the human brain employs two different (and often conflicting) systems to process information and drive decisions and behavior.[2] One system uses logic (*I'll stick to my diet because it's good for me and I've only got ten pounds to lose*), while the other system uses emotion (*I'll eat these chips because they taste so good*). The logic-based system is slow and effortful. It is also where our willpower resides—and, inevitably, exhausts itself. Meanwhile, the emotion-focused system is experiential, nonverbal, and fast. It also motivates us effortlessly, based on our feelings and often outside our awareness.[3] It's no surprise that these very different systems often send us conflicting messages.[4] Even when logic is screaming at you to stay on your diet, you're enjoying those chips before you know what happened.* This understanding goes way beyond dieting, and it applies big time to exercise. If you want to change your behavior in ways you'll sustain, it's very important to understand that our feelings tend to trump logic and the specific outcomes we hope for "in theory."

Research published in the *Journal of Consumer Research* investigated whether people rely more on their *feelings* about an outcome from a choice than *the function of that outcome* in their actual decision making in the moment.[5] Although this study was not about exercising, the findings certainly apply. The closer the impending outcome is to the point of decision, the more people rely on their feelings about it than they do about its ultimate value. For example, consider the action of taking time after work to go to a spinning class. At the moment of leaving work for the class, how you feel about being at the class (looking forward to it or dreading it) more strongly dictates your choice to actually attend than the value of going to the class (it may help you in your quest to lose ten pounds). If you don't enjoy that extreme workout, you are unlikely to stay motivated to go, despite really wanting to lose weight.

In general, human beings approach things that feel good and avoid things that feel bad. This and other research strongly suggests that we must care deeply about how being physically active *makes us feel* if we hope to sustain a lifetime of it.[6] Simply becoming aware of this basic fact gives us the power to make choices about how we move that will set us up for success instead of failure.

---

* For an excellent and very friendly read on these two systems, see Chip Heath and Dan Heath, *Switch: How to Change Things When Change Is Hard* (New York: Broadway Books, 2010).

IT'S YOUR MOVE
Do You Have Negative Feelings
About Physical Exercise?

Before we look more closely at the positive feelings physical activity can generate, take a moment to explore any negative feelings you have in your relationship to exercise:

» In general, when you think about being physically active, do you feel dread?

» Do you feel that there is a "right" way to exercise and that if you don't do it that way, it's not worth doing?

» Do you exercise in ways that don't feel good to you?

High-Intensity Exercise Feels Bad
to a Lot of Folks

You are much more likely to be successful at sustaining high-intensity activity for life if you personally experience it as something positive or at least tolerable. Many people, however, have never felt good from working out vigorously—not even once. And despite a widespread general (though unfounded) belief that if you work out really hard you'll get an endorphin rush, a fascinating body of research by leading exercise psychologist Panteleimon Ekkekakis and his colleagues shows that high-intensity exercise actually tends to *decrease* pleasant feelings.

For more than two decades, Ekkekakis has been studying the

impact of differing exercise intensities on how people feel while they are exercising.[7] This important research shows that there is an inverse relationship between how intensely we exercise and how we feel that follows a dose-response pattern. In other words, the harder someone exercises, the more his pleasure decreases.

Ekkekakis has also found that when people exercise at intensities exceeding the "ventilatory threshold"—that is, the point at which it becomes hard to hold a conversation without panting—not only do they feel less pleasure but they also begin to experience displeasure.[8] This can be highly demotivating. If intense exercise increases negative feelings and decreases positive ones, then you'll be much less likely to keep it up beyond your initial burst of motivation. Why keep doing the workout if you're just going to feel worse? Given the results of this significant program of research, you can begin to see why "no pain, no gain" exercise routines are so difficult to stick to.

Ignoring Your Body Undermines Your Goals

A few years ago, Malia told me that she disdained everything about exercising. When she told me the ways she chose to move, I immediately understood why.

"Every New Year's I commit myself to losing the thirty-seven pounds I've put on since I had my kids," she said. "I join a gym and go at it with a frenzy. I do twenty minutes of stepping as hard and fast as I can, I jump on the treadmill for another thirty minutes, and then I end with ten minutes of rowing."

"And how does that feel to you, Malia?

"Are you kidding, Michelle? I hate every minute of it."

"How long do you keep it up?

"I usually make it to about three weeks."

Malia's story might resonate with you. This is how most people think they have to exercise. But as we learned from the research done by Ekkekakis and his colleagues, high-intensity exercise tends to increase displeasure. Given what we know about what drives our decisions, if high-intensity exercise doesn't feel good to you but you do it anyway, you are not likely to choose to do it consistently.

"Malia," I said, "I'm going to propose a radical idea. How about trying to move in ways that actually feel good to you when you're doing it?"

"But I won't get the benefits if it doesn't hurt to do it!" she exclaimed.

Sadly, most people I've come across still believe this outdated view of exercise. My response is always the same: "How much of those benefits are you getting from doing it three weeks out of the year?" It's hard to argue with reality.

"Not many," she said, defeated.

IT'S YOUR MOVE
Positive and Negative Feelings About Specific Physical Activities

Beginning to see exercise as a gift rather than a chore means drawing on positive experiences and creating new, more motivating Meanings. Even if you are thoroughly in the chore camp right now, you might be surprised to discover that you have actually had at least one good exercise moment that you've forgotten about until now.

Mark below whether you have had positive or negative feelings about the following types of physical activities. If you have a specific memory (e.g., "the way the leaves smelled so fresh when I walked in the forest"), write it down.

ACTIVITY TYPE	POSITIVE	NEGATIVE
Gym class		
Team sports like soccer		
Individual sports like tennis		
Exercising at clubs		
Walking with a friend		
Walking outside		
Walking your dog		
Walking on a treadmill		
Walking on a treadmill watching something		
Walking on a treadmill listening to music you like		
Daily living physical activities (e.g., parking further away, walking to do errands)		
Dancing		
Using home exercise equipment		
Group exercise (Jazzercise, Zumba, etc.)		
Exercising while watching a video at home		
Jumping rope		
Dancing		
Ice skating		
Pilates		
Yoga		
Other		

Did you start to see any patterns in how some physical activities made you feel? It's important for you to start noticing how you feel during these and any other physical activities you could potentially do. Also, notice whether you feel differently about an activity depending on *where* you do it (walking outside versus indoors on a treadmill), *how* you do it (treadmill only versus while listening to music), and with *whom* you do it (alone versus with others). All of these differences influence the experience of moving. It's important for you to start figuring out which experiences feel good and which ones feel bad.

How Autonomy Can Change Your Experience

In stark contrast to Malia, Gina Kolata, fitness writer for the *New York Times*, celebrates her love of working out to the max. In her book *Ultimate Fitness*, she writes, "I discovered that if I work out really hard and for at least forty minutes, I can sometimes reach an almost indescribable state of sheer exhilaration."[9] Some people, like Kolata, swear by their high-intensity workouts. They run marathons, they go on hundred-mile bike rides up steep grades, and they fill the time in between with grueling, sweat-dripping training sessions. I have a number of friends and clients who love to exercise in very intense ways, pushing their bodies to see how far they can go and loving every minute of it. So how is it that they can like this type of hardcore effort when some of us can't stand it?

Although Ekkekakis's research found that people tend to have more displeasure with higher intensity exercise, there is another key finding: When people *decide on their own* to exercise at high intensities, they tolerate it better and experience less displeasure compared to when higher intensity exercise is *imposed on* them.[10] When we *autonomously* choose to exercise at higher intensities, our feelings about our physical activity are not undermined. Why? Because we are choosing to exercise in this way with self-determination, rather than letting pressure or *shoulds* determine our activity choices. Other research agrees: Move in ways that feel good to *you*, whatever that means, and you'll be more physically active over time.[11]

IT'S YOUR MOVE
Your Physical Activities and
Why You Choose Them

Our perception of any behavior as either a chore or a gift has a powerful influence on how we feel about that behavior and, most importantly, on whether we stay motivated to choose it in the moment. Before we move on, I'd like you to take a moment to dig a little deeper into your choices. In the chart below, in the first column, make a list of the physical activities that you've most tended to choose. Then note, in the next column, write the reasons why you've picked those specific activities.

I usually choose the following physical activities for my exercise:

PHYSICAL ACTIVITY	WHY YOU CHOSE IT

The Relationship Between Enjoying Exercise and Losing and Maintaining Weight

An often-cited long-term study conducted in the lab of Pedro J. Teixeira, director of the Physical Activity, Nutrition, and Obesity (PANO) group at the University of Lisbon in Portugal, underscores the tenets of self-determination theory: If you want to be successful over time, you need to take ownership of your exercise and be active in ways that feel good to you.

Teixeira and his colleagues studied a group of overweight women to investigate what kind of motivation was most effective for exercise, weight loss, and maintaining the weight loss over three years.[12] The authors found that feeling greater ownership toward exercise (that is, autonomy) and having more internal reasons to be active (enjoying exercise) were associated with long-term behavior change, but that controlling forms of motivation (*shoulds*) were not. They also found that learning how to enjoy exercise was among the strongest predictors of exercising and maintaining weight loss three years later!

Based on these findings, the authors suggest (and I heartily concur) that programs aiming to create long-term change should abandon pressure and external contingencies (such as imposing punishing financial incentives). Instead, they say, these programs should foster autonomy and internal motivation by helping people own their behavioral choices, find personal significance in their choices beyond behavior change (for example, exercising to lift your mood so you can better enjoy work), and learn how to become physically active in ways that feel good to do. In fact, they believe, these are among the best indicators of whether people will revert to their old habits or move toward adopting an energetic, physically active, and healthy lifestyle.

The implications of this study are profound: When we choose to make movement a regular part of our lives for personally compelling reasons, as well as choosing to move in ways that feel good to us, we are more likely to exercise and also to maintain any weight we lose. It's counterintuitive, right? If you actually want to lose weight that you can keep off over time, stop making your behavioral choices subservient to your weight loss goal. Go beyond weight loss to your daily needs and to what matters most. Many of my clients have told me a similar story: Once they replaced their weight loss goals with a focus on nurturing themselves through their choices about physical activity and eating, the weight comes off without their even trying.

Take ownership of your behavior, make it meaningful, and especially make sure it feels good to you.

It's hard to let go of socialization and what we've been taught by society and those around us. The messages are deeply ingrained within our sense of self. My MAPS program was designed specifically to address the entrenched nature of our Meaning of exercise, and the accumulation of beliefs, feelings, experiences, and reasons that has created this Meaning. Developing a keen Awareness about how our own Meaning has come to be is an essential component of this process.

Illuminating Invisible Chains

I will never forget my client Andy's story about coming face-to-face with the origins of his Meaning for exercise. He was so excited the words just spilled out.

"Michelle," he said, "I was answering the homework questions you gave me last week, and I was completely blown away. When I wrote down the Meaning that exercise had for me, I didn't even have to think about it: punishment. And then this image from when I was a kid just popped into my head." He told me that his dad had been in the military, and his family had traveled all over the world while he was growing up. But no matter where they were living, when he and his siblings misbehaved, her dad would punish them by finding a track and forcing them to run around it until they fell to the ground, exhausted and crying.

"No wonder I think exercise is punishment," he said. "For me and my brothers, it *was* punishment—literally!"

Andy's Meaning for physical activity had been embedded and reinforced early on, and at its core it symbolized punishment. His sudden, vivid insight had an instantaneous effect on his thinking: Illuminating these invisible shackles actually liberated him from their controlling perceptions about exercising. If we are not aware of these deeper Meanings and what caused them, they lurk under every attempt we make to become more physically active and undermine our motivation without our even realizing it. The specific and punitive Meaning Andy had developed of exercise is more dramatic than that of most of my clients. But regardless of what your Meaning is, it's important for you to develop Awareness about it, especially how it came to be.

The process of transforming your Meaning of exercise from a chore to a gift takes more than a moment, but the process is systematic. If you follow my lead, you can easily resocialize yourself toward a lifetime of pleasure-based, personally compelling physical movement. The next step in this journey is excavating the old foundation by doing what I call "exorcising exercise."

How to Exorcise Exercise

Malia and I were having a consultation over the phone when I got to this point in the program with her. I told her, "The next step can feel slightly scary, but it's crucial if you eventually want to change your Meaning of exercise from a chore into a gift."

"Okay," she said, "what do I need to do?"

"Get a piece of paper and a pencil. Then I want you to spend a couple of minutes honestly assessing your most central feelings and beliefs about how you should be exercising, and your expectations and hopes for what exercise is going to do to your body." I gave her time, and then I asked her what she wrote down. She read me the following list:

> » I have to exercise for at least thirty minutes at a time.

> » If I were able to maintain my motivation to exercise, I would be as thin as I was in my twenties.

> » Exercise doesn't count unless I push myself to the limit.

» I have to exercise in a gym or it doesn't count.

» Walking isn't good enough.

After she read the list, I asked, "Malia, do these beliefs and expectations lead you to stay motivated to exercise?"

"No."

"Do they set you up to get pleasure from being active?"

"No."

We talked about how her feelings and expectations had been undermining her desire to sustain a physically active life. Words and thoughts rushed out of her mouth, as if a dam had broken.

Finally, I said, "Now it's time to exorcise exercise. Write down all of your beliefs and expectations that you feel ready to get rid of. After all, if they're not serving you, why would you want to keep them?"

She wrote furiously. When she was done, I said, "Ready? Rip up that paper, Malia!"

I could hear the sounds of tearing over the phone, and I smiled. This activity is a pivotal step in the process of taking ownership over physical activity and converting it from a chore into the gift of a lifetime. Malia had taken that step.

IT'S YOUR MOVE
Exorcise Exercise

Are you ready to toss out the things that have been undermining your motivation and daily decision making, preventing you from the outcomes you deeply desire? This is your opportunity to bring to the surface the old beliefs and expectations, and the Whys that you now know have been preventing you from staying motivated to move your body—especially those that have driven you to choose physical activities that sap you instead of energize you.

This can be a formidable task because it involves rejecting what "experts" and marketers have been teaching you is true. But after so many years of trying something in the same way and getting the same negative results, maybe it's time to try a different approach.

Are you ready to take the driver's seat and remove the pieces that have been getting in your way? If this feels too scary, skip this exercise for now and read more. But consider coming back after you've made it through Chapters 7 and 8, on Permission.

If you do feel ready now, get a piece of paper and a pen or pencil. Set aside two to five minutes, but take as much time as you need to do this assessment.

Start by considering your limiting beliefs or expectations, and write them on the paper. This is an inventory of the beliefs you feel ready to toss out because they have been leading you to fail and feel bad about yourself instead of to succeed and take care of yourself. When you've written them all down and can't think of any more, review your list. If you want to add more undermining beliefs, do so now. If you want to remove something, go ahead.

Ready? Now *rip up the paper and throw it away!*

Some of my clients say that they feel a sudden surge of power when they tear the list to pieces. Others report that they don't feel ready to rip up their list yet or that they want to tape it up as a reminder of what hasn't worked for them so they can mindfully choose things that do. Do what feels right for you.

Exorcising exercise is more than a metaphor. When you exorcise exercise, even if you don't tear up your list, it means you are taking responsibility for what you now know sets you up to fail. Up to this point, these issues were likely not obvious to you because socialization is an unconscious process. It took a lifetime to get to this point. When you participate in this activity, you dig up the beliefs and expectations that have been undermining your own self-care, health, and well being and you shine a light on them. Then, you can eliminate them from your mindset. By doing this, you create space for new beliefs and expectations about physical movement and self-care that will work for you instead of against you.

In the next chapter, you'll learn about the many other ways you can move and the scientific research that gives us the green light to broaden our definition of "what counts." We can expand the number of alternatives available to us every day, making it much easier to sustain an active lifestyle.

The Takeaways

- Being physically active in ways that feel bad to you turns your Meaning for exercise into "a chore."

- When your Whys for exercising are body shaping or achieving weight loss, it frequently leads you to exercise at higher intensities even if you don't like to exercise that way because your objective is to burn as many calories as possible.

- People tend to approach things that feel good and avoid things that feel bad. Your decisions *in the moment* are based on your feelings about an outcome rather than its value to you. So how you feel about an activity (e.g., *How do I feel while I exercise?*) is more likely to determine whether you consistently decide to do it, rather than its value to you (e.g., *How much weight can I lose from this exercise?*).

- In general, when people exercise at intensities past the point at which it becomes hard to hold a conversation without panting, they feel less pleasure and begin to experience displeasure. This dip in pleasure and increase in displeasure can be highly demotivating.

- When people *decide on their own* to exercise at high intensities, they tolerate it better, if not enjoy it, and experience less displeasure compared to when higher-intensity exercise is *imposed* on them by others or *shoulds*. When you *autonomously* choose to exercise at higher intensities, your feelings about your physical activity are not undermined.

- Research shows that when you choose to make movement a regular part of your life for personally compelling reasons and choose to move in ways that feel good to you, you are more likely to stick with exercise and to maintain weight loss.

- In order to change exercise from a chore into a gift, you need to "exorcise" it—to get rid of all of the beliefs, expectations, and Wrong Whys that have been undermining your relationship with movement and your motivation to move.

5

Count Everything and Choose to Move!

TONI CAME TO HER SECOND COACHING SESSION REALLY DISAPPOINTED with herself. She told me, "I missed the exercise class I signed up for because of last-minute work needs. I'm never going to be successful doing this."

Of course, I was curious to learn exactly what had happened. These types of situations provide the clues for understanding what is really getting in a client's way. "What happened?" I asked.

"Well, right when it was time to leave for my class, as per usual, my boss shot me an email with a quick turnaround task. It took only ten minutes to finish, but I didn't have enough time to get to my class."

"Toni, let me understand this more fully. Because you had to do a task that took ten minutes, you didn't have time to make your exercise class. Is that right?"

"Yes, exactly! It takes five minutes to drive to class and five minutes to change. So I would have missed the first ten minutes."

"But didn't you still have thirty minutes left in that class? Why didn't you just get there late?"

She seemed very confused. "How can I go late? I won't get the full workout. I'd miss the beginning . . . " She shook her head. "No, it was too late."

"Toni, most of the time you had allocated to exercise was still available to you. Why didn't you just get what you could out of it?"

"But I missed the full class. It wouldn't have counted!"

I hear this response from virtually all of my clients in the beginning. It reflects what I consider to be the greatest challenge to maintaining a lifetime of physical activity: ideas about what counts and what doesn't count. But it is also a window of opportunity for me to change their thinking on this fundamental misunderstanding.

What "Counts" Is Different from What You Think

For many years, the predominant approach to and recommendation for physical fitness and health was extremely specific and rigid. In fact, it was based on a dose-response equation: Take a *large* amount of specific exercise at *high* intensity to receive optimal health benefits.

Does that seem like the right way to exercise to you? Most people would agree with this idea, but there's new research that expands what "counts."

Around the same time that I began coaching, in 1996, a report came out with a new physical activity recommendation. The report of the U.S. Surgeon General on *Physical Activity and Health* drastically changed what "counted" as exercise and physical activity.[1] Instead of being limited to the old, stringent, one-size-fits-all prescription, this updated recommendation gave us the green light to:

» Accumulate physical activity throughout the day—exercise doesn't have to be done in a single long bout.

» Do activities in less intense ways—physical activity doesn't have to be "vigorous" or make you sweat or breathe extremely hard to count.

» Count as exercise the activities we do naturally during our daily life—including walking, house cleaning, and gardening.

This report told the world that we can gain important health and wellness benefits from engaging in a wider variety of physical activities, intensities, and durations of time than we previously believed. It completely changed the conversation about what counts and what is worth doing. But getting people to believe it, even today, is an uphill battle, and some twenty years after the report came out, most people have not gotten the message. Why? One reason, I think, is a misunderstanding of what I call the ten-minute rule.

The Misunderstood Ten-Minute Rule

If you think that you must do *at least* ten minutes of physical movement in order to benefit, your belief is most likely based on what I consider to be the unfortunate wording of a clarification in the 2007 update to the 1996 report. This recommendation for aerobic activity encouraged people to engage in thirty minutes of moderate-intensity activity five days per week or ten minutes of vigorous intensity activity three days per week, which could be divided up, providing that each instance consisted of at least ten minutes. You can read the entire statement from the American College of Sports Medicine and the American Heart Association,[2] but this is the relevant text:

Clarification in 2007: However, moderate- or vigorous-intensity activities performed as a part of daily life and performed in bouts of 10 minutes or more can be counted toward the recommendation.

The update concludes that the guidelines presented are minimum requirements for preventing disease and strongly encourages American adults to strive for greater amounts of physical activity to gain advanced protection against [inactivity-related chronic disease]. This ten-minute specification remains true through the publication date of this book, so I want to explain why I am concerned.

Right away, I noticed that in the official publication there was no reference or citation next to the ten-minute clarification. I dug a little deeper to find out where the 2007 clarification about the ten minutes came from, and here's what I learned: The 1995 recommendations[3] say that the bouts of activity should be at least eight to ten minutes in duration to be beneficial. This was based on the existing measurement methods at that time. In fact, though, *the research did not show that bouts lasting less than eight minutes did not benefit health.* Rather, the scientific measurement methods of that time could not accurately assess durations of less than eight minutes.

That's an important difference! The recommendation that "activity must be at least ten minutes in duration to count" inadvertently implies that less than ten minutes is not beneficial. Yet scientists—at that time—simply didn't have the tools to accurately assess shorter periods of time. Because the recommendations had to be based on evidence, and the accumulated body of evidence showed that more than ten minutes did benefit health, the authors of the 2007 update were constrained as to what they could say.

I've spoken with many leading scientists in this area and they have told me that they personally believe that bouts of activity shorter than ten minutes provide health benefits but that they didn't have data to support it at the time. I respect their professional restraint. But as a professional who cares about communicating in ways that lead to optimal motivation, participation levels, and sustainability, I believe it would have been better for the official recommendation to explicitly acknowledge that this ten-minute clarification was based on findings that at least eight to ten consecutive minutes of exercise did have health benefits, but was *not* based on evidence showing that activity of less than eight to ten minutes did not benefit health.

Since the 2007 update was published, there has been a growing body of research using new wearable technologies, such as activity trackers (Jawbone Up, Fit Smart, Fitbit, etc.), which can measure periods of activity of less than eight minutes. Some of the findings emerging out of this newer research suggest that activity bouts of less than ten minutes also contribute toward positive markers of health,[4] in addition to other immediately noticeable perks such as boosting energy and mood.[5]

This research is still in its infancy, so there are no definitive answers yet. However, research that too much sitting is bad for our health further suggests that having a ten-minute guideline for activity might be shooting ourselves in the foot.

Sitting May Be Bad for Your Health

Marc Hamilton, at the Pennington Biomedical Research Center, studies the effects of sedentary behavior—sitting, lying on the couch, not moving—on physiology. His research shows that inactive time undermines cardiovascular and metabolic health.[6] Hamilton and others suggest we might consider inactivity as a serious health hazard, on a par with smoking when it comes to health risks. He calls for updated physical activity and health guidelines to include recommendations that address too much sitting time.[7] His work would suggest that we don't need sweat-producing, heavy-breathing exercise to get real physiological benefits—just regular ole body movement will do.

The idea that sitting less can improve our health is further supported by other research on the effects of movement on the length of telomeres, the caps on the end of DNA that protect our chromosomes and are physiological markers of health and longevity. (Shorter telomeres indicate aging and illness; longer ones indicate better health.) Telomere length, physical activity, and sitting time were measured at the beginning of a physical activity intervention in sedentary, overweight individuals in their late sixties and then six months later. The findings are counterintuitive and compelling. Reduced sitting time over the six months was associated with longer telomere length, indicating better health. In contrast, time spent in more formal exercise was negatively associated with telomere length. The takeaway from this study was that sitting less had positive effects on telomere length while exercising did not.[8]

These studies, combined with the established science showing that some of the physiological benefits that we gain from physical activity (for example, those related to preventing and managing type 2 diabetes) *quickly* decline after exercising,[9] underscores the importance of moving *consistently* and *frequently* during our daily life.

Which brings us back to the ten-minute rule and my concerns about it. One of the most important reasons why I do not advocate the ten-minute rule is this: It leads people to choose *not* to move when they have less than ten minutes because they don't think it will "count." That adds up to a whole lot of minutes that could have been used to move but weren't.

A prescription for lifestyle change to optimize health seems like good medicine. But if most people are not motivated to sustain it over time, then the actual health benefits will be small. Establishing a threshold for movement allows for only two options: success or failure. When people believe they must achieve a specific target in order to make movement worthwhile—whether it's ten minutes or twenty minutes or forty-five minutes—their restricted definition of what success looks like actually thwarts their ability to successfully stick with it when life throws a curveball. This is just like what happened with Toni.

IT'S YOUR MOVE
Check Your Beliefs About What Counts

Remember the exercise in Chapter 1 where you considered what "counts" as exercise and is worth doing? Think about how you answered those questions then. Now, consider the questions below again in light of what you read in this chapter. Would you answer them any differently?

1. In general, for exercise to "count" or be worth doing, I have to do it for _____ minutes at a time.

2. In general, *before reading this book,* I believed that for physical movement to be worth doing, I needed to (circle one):

   Breathe hard and sweat

   Move

To Sweat or Not to Sweat?

If you are like most people I've spoken to for the last two decades—including most fitness and medical professionals—you chose "breathe hard and sweat" for your answer to the second question above. That answer reflects the predominant socialization virtually everyone today has had regarding the "right" way to be physically active.

Yet I'm suggesting that movement itself—not necessarily high-intensity, work-up-a-dripping-sweat movement—is the most important thing for you to do if you don't like intense exercise and the "hard and sweaty" recommendation has not worked for you long term. I know this can be confusing, so let me take a moment to clarify.

I am not saying that moving in ways that promote sweating and hard breathing is wrong or that this shouldn't be your objective. Research shows that, in general, the more physical movement you do, the greater your health benefits will be,[10] within reason. And I am all for movement and health!

One more thing: You are not being lazy if you don't work up a sweat. The casual use of the word *lazy* always concerns me, because calling ourselves lazy as an explanation for not taking care of ourselves or moving our bodies actually undermines our motivation and self-respect, as you'll learn in Chapter 10. What's really going on?

First, people can mistake being just plain tired for laziness. Most of us these days are worn out simply from the amount of juggling we have to do in our lives. At the end of a hard day we just want to relax and decompress—which is a valid response, and very different from being "lazy." Just thinking about how much we actually have to do in any given day can be exhausting and overwhelming.

And there's another very important issue here. It's pretty easy to conclude that we're lazy when we hold ourselves to an unrealistic (or outdated) "gold standard" of physical activity. The more moderate physical fitness recommendations have been around for almost two decades. Despite this, the messages from older recommendations as well as the marketing from fitness companies are hard to override and still lead many people to believe that *real* exercise has to be hard and vigorous, and that only a certain kind of workout for a set duration of time (no pain, no gain) is of benefit. It's hard *not* to buy into a societal ideal for physical activity and exercise that is everywhere—on billboards, on television, on the Internet, in the movies, in magazines, even from our trusted healthcare providers. On top of that, when we see some of our friends doing hard workouts four days a week or training for marathons, our realization that we can't do what they're doing (or don't want to do it) just confirms our suspicion about ourselves.

But believing that we are lazy is not only a very self-deprecating way to think about why we are choosing not to move. It's bad for our motivation, and it also stands between us and a whole world of movement choices and possibilities. It's discouraging to work past your comfort zone, especially when you are still at the beginning of establishing an enjoyable relationship with movement. Most people don't stay motivated to exercise when they dislike the activity, dislike how it makes them feel, or can't find a way to fit it into their overly scheduled lives. That's a normal, human response. It's not a personality flaw.

The goal I'm suggesting is much larger than piling up hours per day and days per week of exercise: I want you to be able to sustain—happily—whatever physical activities you choose to do over your lifetime, and I want those activities to provide consistent energy for all of the other parts of your complex, wonderful life.

So lazy, schmazy! You are still going to get benefits from your physical activities *if you choose to move in ways you like and that fit into your day*. Anything is better than nothing, period.

When it comes to creating a lifetime of movement, we need to step outside the laboratory and into real life. It's okay to look outside the gym for opportunities to move. I am not saying exercise is not good for your health. (It is.) And I am not saying that you should not follow your medical professional's suggestion to get more exercise. (Of course you should!) I am saying that the medical model of exercise—the paradigm itself—doesn't work for most people. Before we move on, I want to make sure you understand why.

Moving Away from the Medical Model of Exercise

"Exercise is medicine" makes sense as a way to persuade clinicians to promote physical activity to their patients. But framing exercise as medicine is not a very compelling metaphor for consistent, long-term participation for many people.

Physical activity prescribed as a "dose" of movement automatically makes us think that physical activity is analogous to taking medicine.* One of the greatest problems with this approach is that the original behavior—getting people to take their medicine—is notorious for low compliance rates around the world.[11] Taking specific pills at specific times during the day is not a simple behavior, but it is still less complicated from a time and logistics standpoint than sustaining a physically active life amid the many other daily calls on our attention.

The medical model of exercise simply doesn't take the realities of real life (and emotionally motivated decision making) into account. First, this approach assumes that the conditions of our lives are sufficiently controllable to permit us to successfully achieve those specific doses of activity. For some, like my husband, it is. But life is unpredictable or at least constantly changing. Despite our best efforts to schedule appointments and keep them, something is bound to come up.

Second, prescribing optimal doses of physical activity assumes that we regularly base our choices on what is in our best interest and that our daily decision making occurs consciously and logically. But as we've seen, the science about decision making shows that these assumptions of rationality and conscious decision making are incorrect: Most of our daily choices occur unconsciously and we frequently don't do what is in our best interest.[12] Even if we didn't have this compelling science about human cognition and decision making, we have one indisputable finding: The old medically based, exercise-based model has not successfully guided most people to sustain physically active lives.

Some medical issues do call for specific physical activity remedies.

---

* A global movement called Exercise Is Medicine (http://exerciseismedicine.org) aims to get healthcare providers to understand the value of prescribing physical activity as literal medicine to patients. While this branding/education campaign makes sense for clinicians, it is not a message that will optimally motivate most individuals to sustain physically active lives, because of the science and behavioral reasons discussed in this book.

For example, cardio work that gets your heart rate up has measurable health benefits for many people and can be a lifesaver for some. But these kinds of traditional physical activities are just one part of a very interesting story that moves us away from the medical model of pre-scribed activity and into a treasure hunt for movement options in real life.

Let's look at a life-centered, real-world fitness model that lets you tailor movement to fit who *you* are and how *you* live, instead of the other way around. Many more of us can become much more consis-tently active if we appreciate the realities of hectic modern living and start to *count everything*.

Everything Counts:
A Better Message to Motivate More Movement

After working with individuals in real life on this issue, I've come to believe that a better message for more consistent physical movement is that we should count any and every opportunity to move that exists in the space of our lives as valid movement worth doing. Some don't agree with me, and occasionally, someone tells me that the idea I'm suggesting that you should count everything is just "dumbing down" the physical activity recommendation. I want to be very clear here:

» I'm *not* saying that if you notice you've been walking in the gro-cery store and to and from your car, then you don't need to move more than that because you are already being "active."

» I *am* saying that you should give yourself credit for what you are already doing. What counts as physical movement *for you* needs to come out of realistic expectations about how you will benefit from doing it, what your personal preferences are for moving your body, and what types of activities you can actu-ally fit in and stick with, given your current life circumstances.

Some medical professionals are concerned that individuals who believe everything they do "counts" will move *less* because they will think that what they are doing already is sufficient. On the surface, that's a legitimate concern. But it ignores a reality that successful marketers are well aware of: If you want people to choose your product or behavior of interest, make it as easy as possible.

The food industry has been exploiting this principle in their marketing strategies for years. Specifically, they aim to facilitate access to food by making it easier to purchase, prepare, and consume.[13] They do everything they can to make a *choice* effortless for consumers, because they've learned that people *want and will choose what's easy*. So food marketers do everything they can to remove barriers at the very point of purchase for consumers. The marketers also already have an asset on their side: We tend to treat eating as a mindless, habitual activity. We're ready to just do it. If a particular food is attractively packaged, we like the taste, we want it right now, and it's readily available . . . we buy it and eat it. No thinking needed.

Now contrast that with the physical activity world. In essence, we've been encouraging people to forgo tasty physical activity "snacks" they can consume any time and instead buy large, expensive, multi-course meals—and they have to get specially dressed to partake of many of those meals. We've created standards and rules for moving that actually make it *more* complicated to move—an activity that is an essential part of life, like eating.

Our goal as physical activity promoters has not been to make movement as easy as possible for everyone. Instead, we've been trying to make sure that people do it "right." But doing it *properly*—that is, doing specific types of exercise for the proper amount of time, in the proper place, and with the proper clothing—often means that it becomes easier for people not to do it at all. (This topic is explored more fully below.)

IT'S YOUR MOVE
Do You *Really* Have No Time?

On days when you are rushing around and feeling as if you have no time to take even one more extra step, let alone fit in some physical activity, ask yourself this: Is it true that you don't have time for one more step? Or is it that you don't have a *full thirty minutes* to spare, so you think it's not worth doing anything at all?

When I ask my clients to consider this question, most are surprised to find it's the latter. You can almost always choose to modify your plans and just move— even if it's only a few more steps.

In contrast, the concept that everything counts converts that hard-to-hit bull's-eye of specific times and techniques into a whole wall of movement options people can do at any time. This mindset motivates people to participate in more physical activity in sustainable ways.[14] Because we can't miss the wall, we are more likely to feel confident about choosing to move whenever we are able. That's crucial, because confidence, or self-efficacy, for physical activity is a very important element to have in place if you hope to maintain it over time.[15]

When we accept this new life-centered way of thinking about physical movement, the world is filled with opportunities to move that we never noticed. Suddenly, we start enjoying the challenge of discovering all sorts of creative and unexpected ways to fit smaller bits of movement into our day, and we give ourselves credit for taking literal strides toward our well-being, health, and fitness—further reinforcing our motivation.

The type of movement available from formal, structured exercise—aerobics classes, spinning, weight training, dance workouts, and all the rest of the classes you can choose from at the gym—is very beneficial, especially if you like doing it. If it's working for you, keep it up. But when everything counts, why limit yourself to *only* going for a run or spending forty minutes on the treadmill? Each day offers a wide and infinitely varied continuum of opportune moments of movement options from which to choose.

Understanding That "Everything Counts" Is a Bridge to Consistency

When I have followed up with clients after some years and asked them about their perceptions of which elements of the program helped them be active and stay active, virtually everyone has told me that the notion that "everything counts" was transformative for them. Deb, one of my earliest clients, came to me nearly twenty years ago, when she was forty-two. Today, she says, "For me, one of the most important concepts from the program was that everything counts: every step, every motion, every action. I learned that no matter how little it is, just keep moving! I missed my exercise class—but anything is better than nothing. If I have only five minutes available, then five minutes it will be."

When we allow all sorts of physical activities and amounts of movement into the mix, it removes the barriers to choosing to move. If everything counts, there is no need to wonder whether this move is worth making or whether it is the proper amount of time to "count." In an "everything counts" mindset, moving can become much *more automatic* because once the opportunity, or cue, to move presents itself, we don't have to engage the cognitive, slow, and effortful system of our brain. Instead, we can just glide into action—because it's there. When we believe that everything counts and that every opportunity to move is a gift we can give ourselves, we are much more likely to seek and claim that gift from the multitude of opportunities we encounter all day long.

The belief that everything counts builds a new bridge from "I don't have time" to "I can fit this in!" It gives some people permission to do a different type of movement on the days they can't do as much as they had planned to do. It gives permission to others who might not be inclined toward or want formal exercise to do an alternative form of movement that might be more palatable and realistic. I've found that "everything counts" leads people to move more and, because of that, they start to consider themselves as physically active individuals. This new sense of identity motivates even more daily movement,[16] which reinforces this new positive identity.

As Mariam, one of my workshop participants, said:

> Once I started paying attention to what I was doing during the day—beyond just sitting at the computer—I was amazed at how much more active I was than I had thought, and really how many more opportunities I had to move just in my office than I was taking. It became a game—oh, I can walk a couple of flights of stairs instead of taking the elevator! I can take a fifteen-minute walk during lunch instead of spending the whole time eating a sandwich at my desk. It sounds like nothing, but it's a lot, and it's actually fun and challenging. I am more conscious of everything I do now, and I seek out all the opportunities for movement I can find. It makes me feel good about myself and energizes me!

It All Adds Up

Please keep doing formal, structured exercise if it works for you, if it benefits you, and if you like it. But if you've struggled and have been discouraged time and again to make that type of movement fit into your life, then how about trying another way? How about considering that every bit of movement you do is adding to your health, fitness, and joie de vivre? Here are some ways to start:

» Try fitting physical activity into your day any way you can. There are lots of ideas in this chapter to get you started.

» Ask your friends, your coworkers, your partner, and your children to join you in short bouts of activity, and explain why it is worth the effort. This will start to create cultures of movement all around you. (This benefits everyone!)

» At the beginning, shoot for finding seven to ten minutes of movement a day, or whatever is realistic for your current life. Try that for a week and then evaluate how easy or difficult it was. Notice if it felt good to move in the way you chose. After you evaluate that, decide if you want to keep it the same, ramp it up, or decrease it if you discovered that was too much for now.

Get creative. Get proactive. Choose to move in whatever ways you can. Incorporate all kinds of physical activity into your life. The idea is to add up the increments—whether it's one half-hour yoga class, several short sessions of walking during the day, or five minutes of walking up and down the stairs plus ten minutes of yard work plus a fifteen-minute walk to pick up a loaf of bread at the store—and aim to do as much as you can.

This is truly about you and *your* life. Take charge and decide what is best for you, today. You are at the beginning of a new path, and it takes time to learn how to do new things. So for now, just experiment. Do what you can. And most importantly, feel good about *everything* that you are able to do!

You can find numerous gifts of movement every day in your own life. You just have to look around to discover where they are.

A Treasure Hunt:
Discovering Hidden Opportunities to Move

Finding opportunities to move (my clients abbreviate this as OTMs, so I will too) throughout the day is surprisingly fun. You'll be amazed at how soon you begin to become aware of the free spaces in the day that present themselves and the surprising places that are conducive to movement. You may think that your day is crammed so full that you can't fit in one more thing, but believe me: It's not true. If you've got one minute, you've got time.

Use the following examples to jump-start your ideas, then enlist the help of your friends, your children, and your partner. I guarantee that every new day will bring at least one new opportunity to move that you have never considered. These examples are given in no particular order, so just dive in. You can start right where you are—no special outfits necessary.

The Long Cut

I wish I'd made this one up, but I have a friend to thank for it. As you probably have already guessed, the Long Cut is the opposite of the shortcut. It means strategically discovering a longer walking route to a destination in order to build in more time to move. You can take the Long Cut anywhere—to work, while you're shopping, and so on. Try parking your car a little further from your destination. You can build in a round-trip of ten or more minutes of movement.

The Phone Moment

When you're talking on your cell phone or cordless phone, get up and walk around. You can take the opportunity to water houseplants, start a meal, feed your pets, go up and down stairs, or even take a walk around the block.

Active Waiting

When kids are playing organized sports, most of their moms and dads are either waiting in the car or sitting around chatting with other parents. Of course, you want to watch your child play some of the time, but you can also use this opportunity to get your own movement time. You can do Active Waiting around the perimeter of a park or track, or if your kids are safe in an indoor class or other sporting situation, you can leave to take a trail or even just walk along the closest street. Always be sure to let your child know your plans and that you may not be present for the entire class or game.

You can do Active Waiting alone or, as I do, plan to walk with another parent. While our sons are in their forty-five-minute karate class, my friend Kim and I sometimes walk for twenty minutes and watch for twenty-five, or we walk for the full class. Sometimes we sit and watch the whole class. We follow the everything-in-moderation philosophy and do what feels right on that day. Discovering this option was a relief for me. It not only gives me an opportune time to move but it gives me time with my friend to share and laugh. Adult conversation can be a great motivator for a parent. I am a different person when we return.

Before we leave Active Waiting, I want to address a common barrier that many parents have at first to this approach: guilt. Parents feel it's their duty to watch their kids learn and excel at a physical activity or sport, and it is. But it's also your duty to take care of yourself and meet your own needs. In addition, research shows that having active parents is key for teaching children that making time to move is a priority and something worth fitting in. Become aware of any guilt you might have and acknowledge it without judgment. Then ask yourself if watching your child for the full time at *every* practice or game is really that superior to watching part of the time, building in time for your movement, and as a bonus modeling that even busy adults can prioritize movement and self-care and strategize ways to fit it in.

The Movement Snack

When you're not quite ready for a meal but your stomach is growling, you reach for a snack to tide you over. You can do exactly the same thing with exercise. When your body is sending the message to move but you don't have the full thirty or forty minutes available, you can still grab a five- or ten-minute refresher. Grab a bite whenever you can!

The Couple's Cruise

It's lovely to walk with your partner and catch up during some alone time. It's much harder, if not impossible, to get away when you have young kids. But if you can switch off with a neighbor or get a sitter, consider dinner and a walking cruise instead of dinner and a movie. Cruising with your partner before or after dinner can be very intimate, a time to spontaneously share, watch people, hold hands, and be together in one of the most basic parts of life—walking.

The Boogie Break

As someone who loves to dance to music from the 1980s (yes, I'm sorry), I can't believe it took until the year I was writing this book to discover this gem. When I need a stretch or simply a break (in the privacy of my office or home), I pick a song, put on earphones, and get down, get down, get down! This is an amazing way to get a lot of energy, loosen up, and lift your mood. Just think Ellen DeGeneres and start dancing!

The Green Getaway

Ahhh. Smell that fresh air! Nature in all its manifestations—from forest, ocean, lake, and mountains to city park, pocket park, or backyard garden—offers a needed escape from the stressors of life, urban rush and noise, and too many screens. Getting out in nature lets you clear your head and start to feel like yourself again. The Green Getaway is a gift to your mental and physical health. Recent research shows time and again that moving our bodies brings incredible benefits in mood and energy. Research also shows that the more you actively look at and engage with green spaces—hills, mountains, trees, grass—the more cognitive, restorative benefits you'll get.[17]

It's a Gift

This is more than finding a way to fit some movement in: It is the time you consciously give yourself to move as an explicit gift to your body, your mind, and your spirit. Any type of physical movement will do. I have some clients who use this time to take a yoga, Pilates, or tai chi class or do something more intense like spinning or Zumba. Other clients prefer to go to the park and walk, run, or bike there, enjoying the changing seasons. Still others go into the city and walk around different neighborhoods and shops. It doesn't matter what you do as long as the activity is just for you and you feel nurtured and refueled by it.

Friend Fitness

Our relationships are among the most meaningful and feel-good parts of living. Moving with friends while walking, biking, or taking a class can create a deeper connection or simply be an enjoyable experience. And there's a bonus: You may have already noticed that you are likely to do your activity for a longer period of time than usual if you are doing it with others.

Family Fun

Finding opportunities to move with your family brings many other rewards along with physical movement. Tossing a ball, chasing each other, playing tag, dancing, swimming, walking, skating—you can do all sorts of activities with family members. Moving with your family is a time for playing, catching up, and simply bonding, and it may be among your family's most treasured memories. Family Fun can be as structured as a bike ride taken together, as raucous as a backyard game of tetherball, or as simple as a leisurely evening walk around the block to transition into nighttime. Also consider pairing up a child and parent. When I was a teenager, my dad and I would run together, both at home and on vacation, and that alone time was a great way for us to bond.

Working Walk or Walking Meeting

Some of my most productive meetings take place while I am walking—either with the other person or while talking with him on the phone. And I'm not alone. Many of my friends and clients report that they have better ideas and feel freed up for creativity when they walk and work outside of the office environment. The keys to effective Walking Meetings (besides avoiding loud traffic) boil down to safety: Stay alert to your surroundings and walk intelligently and defensively (watching out for cars, cyclists, and other walkers). If you need to take notes on your call, you can record the call with an app or take voice notes.

Recess

It's not just for kids! This is something a lot people do without thinking of it as fulfilling an exercise requirement: getting together with friends to run, hike, skate, or play hoops, handball, tennis, ping-pong, softball, field hockey, soccer, or flag football.

The Soulful Stroll

When you are feeling down or melancholy and you just need to connect with your feelings in a self-compassionate, nonjudgmental way, adding movement can be a tremendous help. Rather than pulling the covers over your head and hibernating, use movement to honor rather than reject what you are feeling. You might want to walk slowly or do something at high intensity, depending on the type of physical feelings that you know you need and want to have.

Coffee Walk

Why sit? Instead of meeting a friend to talk at a café, grab your coffee or tea to go and head out to enjoy the outdoor setting while you catch up and window-shop.

Doggy Destinations

Several of my animal-friendly clients told me that they originally got a dog to create the daily need to take them for walks, thus getting a walk themselves. You can be the leader or let your dog's nose find new places for you to go. Just make sure to bring a baggy with you.

Office Sprints

The office, which seems practically dedicated to sitting, actually offers some easy ways to add movement to your day. Instead of eating lunch at your desk, go for a walk outside, find a park or a bench, and eat your lunch there. Get up from your chair and stretch periodically. Instead of taking the elevator, take the stairs. Or just use the stairs as an in-house gym for a few minutes any time you feel like a break. Instead of sitting at your desk, try standing up and working. Standing desks—and even very, very slow treadmills to use while standing and working—are now becoming a popular option in a number of offices. While it's not for me, many of my friends and colleagues love them!

Cleaning Calisthenics

Anyone who has ever pushed a vacuum cleaner knows that it provides exercise. Household chores count as valid physical movement, so take advantage of the opportunities doing them can present. For example, you can build in additional trips to the laundry room, carrying smaller loads to get more movement in. Count yourself lucky if you have stairs in your house!

Be a Sport

I know many middle-aged adults who've returned to sports they enjoyed as kids or decided to try sports for the first time. A colleague of mine started doing field hockey, my sister decided to learn tae kwon do and is now hooked, one of my clients joined a masters swimming program at the YMCA, and almost every workplace has a softball league.

Gym Genius

Although this book has stressed moving beyond the idea that you need a gym in order to exercise, it's no surprise that gyms and fitness clubs are a great place to find more structured types of movement like classes or workouts using machines, weights, swimming pools, and other apparatus. If you attend a gym where you feel welcomed and comfortable, this can be a wonderful way to feed your spirit on your own terms or to connect with a community of people while you work out. What you do is up to you. I have found that people understand when I honestly say, "I'd really love to talk with you now but I only have twenty minutes to fit in my workout before I have to go." Or you could say, "I'd love to talk. Want to grab the treadmill next to mine?"

The Leisurely Stroll

Europeans tend to include what we think of exercise as a basic part of daily life. When I lived in Barcelona, my friend Roser would regularly call me up and ask, "Quieres pasiar?" She was asking if I felt like taking a stroll down the lovely Las Rambles boulevard with her. Strolling for fun—not power-walking, not counting the blocks or tracking your mileage, just enjoying the walk—is relaxing, great exercise and a totally underappreciated activity that you can do alone or with others.

Walk the Airport

You're going to be sitting on that plane for hours, right? Why start early? Instead of sitting and working while you're waiting to board your plane, take some of that time to walk around with your wheeled luggage (or store it for an hour if you have time).

Airplane Activity

You don't have to remain seated when the seatbelt sign is off, so take opportunities to move when they present themselves: Walk the length of the plane or stand in the back and do calf raises. You'll find a small but dedicated community of plane walkers sharing smiles with you. If you want to remain seated, do seated stretches.

One-Minute Workout

All of us have at least one extra minute in our day. When you have one, use it to do whatever movement feels best and most convenient at that moment: Walk up and down stairs, do jumping jacks, stand up and sit down, do your favorite yoga pose, stretch . . . it's your choice! Remember, it all adds up.

The Snow Shuffle

I owe this idea to a client who was working on ways she could walk to work without breaking her neck in the sometimes treacherous Michigan snow and ice. She discovered shoe "chains" (yes, like tire chains for shoes) in a local sporting goods store, and she has never let winter stop her from walking since.

IT'S YOUR MOVE
Find an Opportunity to Move

If you've been sitting and reading this chapter for a while, it's time to get up out of your chair and find an opportunity to move. Take a few minutes to move your body and refresh your mind before moving on to the next chapter.

When everything counts, you can discover an infinite number of valid and worthwhile ways to integrate physical activity into your busy life. The many gifts of movement are indeed everywhere. In the next chapter, you'll learn how you can transform exercise from a chore into the gift that you'll want to give yourself every day as many times as you like.

The Takeaways

- The updated, more moderate physical activity recommendations (from 1996 and 2007) expand the definition of what type of physical movement people can do every day: You can accumulate exercise, do it at lower intensities, and count life-centered activities like housework and gardening.

- The update that the duration of physical activity needs to be at least ten minutes long to benefit health was based on not having methods sophisticated enough to measure physical activity that was less than eight minutes long. There is growing support, using advanced measurement technologies, that shorter amounts of movement can benefit health and energy levels, and that being sedentary promotes physiological changes that harm health.

• The medical model of exercise has not worked for most people over the last thirty years. By contrast, life-centered fitness—where all of the activities of daily life count in addition to structured gym activities—is everywhere and accessible to everyone all day long.

• What counts as physical movement—for you—needs to come out of realistic expectations about how you will benefit from doing it, what your personal preferences are for moving your body, and what types of activities you can actually sustain over time, given your life circumstances.

• Once you start to believe that everything counts, you'll see that every day offers a wide and infinitely varied continuum of opportunities to move (OTMs) that you can choose to take advantage of anytime. Deciding to believe that everything counts can be your bridge to building consistent daily movement that you can immediately benefit from.

• An important step toward embracing movement in your life is simply to become aware that your choices about how you move through your day truly are *your choices*.

• Finding OTMs is a treasure hunt! The OTMs presented in this chapter are examples of the many ways you can gift yourself movement throughout your day.

6

From a Chore to a Gift

I WORKED WITH LAILA ALMOST FOUR YEARS AGO. SHE'D BEEN LEADING a sedentary life—busy at her desk all day at work, sitting in front of the TV at night. At our first meeting, she told me, "I feel like a slug." She said that she wanted to "get back in shape," but she was downright negative about her options. She didn't like the gym (too much trouble), she didn't like running (the pounding hurt her knees), she didn't like riding a bike (she could never master the gears and going uphill was too hard), and she didn't like skiing or snowboarding (the idea of sliding down an icy slope on flat sticks seemed crazy). Her list was long and her resistance was strong.

"I was at the point where I felt apathetic about exercise and victimized by not being able to stick with it over time, and I called you," she reflected. "At first, I thought your ideas were touchy-feely, and I was hesitant to trust you. But when I did the exorcising exercise and realized that I wrote down *I hate exercise*, I thought, yeah, I hate it, and that's why I'm here. Once I let myself start to think about the beliefs that had been driving my decisions and choices and saw them on paper, it was a shock. I realized that I couldn't stick my head in the sand and just ignore them anymore."

Laila's list included the convictions that only "traditional" exercise counted, that she had to work out at the gym, and that her workouts had to be "serious." When she wrote these beliefs down on paper and saw them staring back at her in black and white, she felt oppressed by them. She knew that they didn't reflect what she wanted for herself. If they did, she wondered, why had she come to me for help in the first place?

With this new Awareness, Laila's resistance began to crumble and she started to feel the swell of new excitement: Maybe she really could do things differently. Maybe things could change.

She tried one new physical activity and then another. As she moved forward, she found new reasons to move, reasons that more directly reflected how she felt on a daily basis. She determined her Right Why (for the time being), and she started moving in ways she liked that energized her day. These positives reinforced each other and converted her Meaning of exercise into a gift—her gift.

Recently, I reconnected with Laila online. She told me that she had been regularly active for the past four years. She had deepened her relationship with physical activity. "That's good to hear," I responded. "What happened?"

"It was exactly what you suggested would happen—that everything would change if I connected with a reason for change that was mine and picked activities that I actually liked to do. Everything did change. It turned out to be inline skating, which I loved as a kid. I started out renting them in the park one afternoon, and I was hooked."

Laila bought new skates, along with a helmet and pads for her knees and elbows. "I was really excited about buying them," she told me. "I hadn't been that happy about doing something physical since I was fifteen. I feel like skating is exactly what my body wants to do. I even tried skating to work. My coworkers probably think I'm crazy, but it's pretty awesome. It's a great way to start the day. I feel like myself for the first time in a long time."

When you move from the Wrong Why to the Right Why, as Laila did, it opens the window to a new world where exercise looks very different than it used to. In that new world, your motivation to move your body comes from yourself rather than from what you think is right, permissible, or allowed. Just realizing that you've been forcing yourself to exercise and that it *feels like a chore* may be all it takes to change everything.

Reframing:
From the Wrong Why to the Right Why

A physical therapist who attended one of my MAPS behavioral sustainability trainings emailed me about a month afterward to tell me an inspiring story about her patient Marla. Marla was sixty-eight and recovering from a stroke. The doctor told her that she needed to do regular facial exercises to counteract the facial droop that resulted from the stroke. But she hated those exercises because she felt they were boring and because every time she did them, it reminded her of the ordeal she'd been through and that her body no longer worked the way she wanted it to. It was frustrating and upsetting and sad for her.

Marla left her physical therapy sessions with the intention to follow her recovery plan, but she just wasn't motivated and even felt a deep-seated resistance to doing the exercises. This conflict between what she had planned to do and what she chose to do is known as the "gap between intentions and behavior." It's a well-accepted phenomenon within healthcare that reflects both our good intentions for taking care of ourselves and a deeper ambivalence we feel about the behavior or prescribed treatment plan.

Marla's physical therapist made an interesting suggestion. "Marla," she said, "instead of thinking about the stroke that's forcing you to do these exercises, think about what you'll gain from doing them. Can you think of a benefit *you'd* like?"

Marla didn't have to think for long: Strengthening her facial muscles would mean she could regain her ability to smile.

"Can you imagine some occasions where you'd really want to be able to smile?" the therapist asked.

"My daughter getting married in August, the birth of my grandchildren . . ." Tears came to her eyes when she talked about it. Clearly, she had found a new, much more meaningful reason to do her exercises. In essence, Marla had replaced a Wrong Why ("because my physical therapist prescribed the exercises for me as part of my recovery") with her own, personalized Right Why ("because I want to smile"), which immediately enabled her to transform the Meaning of the exercises from a chore into a gift. Once Marla created a deeply personal reason—her Right Why—for doing the exercises, she discovered that she was motivated to make them a priority.

At this point, you might be wondering what your Right Why might be. If you're ready to start considering which of the many amazing reasons to move your body is *your* Right Why, allow me to present some of the many Whys that may inspire you.

Many Right Whys:
Regular Physical Activity Is an Elixir of Life

In the ancient world, East and West, philosophers and explorers sought the elixir of life, the mythical potion said to bring eternal youth and life. They never found it, but we have the next best thing right now: Physical activity truly is a real-world elixir of life, and it brings an abundance of mind-body-spirit benefits.

What your Right Why is depends on what you need right now. But the following *It's Your Move* exercise offers you a chance to explore many different evidence-based benefits from moving,[1] just some of many potential Right Whys that can help you live better and feel better today.*

---

* To dive deep into the ways exercising changes our brain so that we feel more joyful and less stressed, read John J. Ratey and Eric Hagerman, *Spark: The Revolutionary New Science of Exercise and the Brain* (New York: Little, Brown and Company, 2008).

IT'S YOUR MOVE
Your Physical Activity Gift List

Put a check mark next to any of the physical activity gifts listed below that you would like to experience. Then, if you're not sure which of these Right Whys is the best one for you right now, I suggest giving the first one—enhancing energy—a test drive.

Your Right Why is not a fixed idea—it's a moving target. As your life changes, your Right Why might also change. Remember, the Right Whys for movement aim to serve you and your life. If and when your life needs different things, reevaluate whether your Why and activity choices are still a good fit.

I NEED MORE ✓	PHYSICAL MOVEMENT CAN ENHANCE . . .	I NEED LESS ✓	PHYSICAL MOVEMENT CAN DECREASE . . .
	Energy		Stress
	Mood		Anxiety
	Life satisfaction		Depression
	Sleep		Cognitive decline
	Productivity		Addictive behavior/ substance abuse (i.e., helps control addictions)
	Sex life		Getting sick all the time (increases immunity)
	Creativity		ADHD
	Executive functioning (e.g., memory, problem solving, control of cognitive processes)		Menopausal symptoms
	Strength for daily activities		PMS
	Self-worth		Low self-esteem

Forget about abstract, distant benefits from moving that you *might* experience in the future and start choosing Whys that offer real, concrete ways to meaningfully enhance the quality of your daily life *now*.

Why Isn't "To Be Healthy" a Right Why?

In my keynotes and behavioral trainings, people inevitably challenge me when I suggest that "health-promoting" Whys are the Wrong Whys. They tell me that health is central to their work or that they care deeply about their health. But for health to be a *real* Right Why, it has to be a real motivator for consistent, ongoing behavior. It has to be a reason for daily decision making that drives you to do it regularly.

Most of us value our health—that's not the issue. The issue is whether "health" is a *strategic* Why for lasting motivation and behavior change. Remember, how we *feel* about exercising is going to be more influential to our decisions in the moment about whether we exercise than the future value of exercising,[2] including "better health." This is "delay discounting" (a phenomenon described in the behavioral economics field), which refers to a general tendency to choose immediate over future rewards.[3] And as much as we'd like to think it's not so, for most people, worrying about having a heart attack in twenty or thirty years is not going to determine if they do their planned morning run or choose to sleep through the alarm today. If "better health" keeps you motivated, then it is a Right Why for you. Only you can make that determination based on your past experiences using better health as your Why.

We'd like to be active to improve our health, but it simply doesn't make physical movement relevant enough for many of us to prioritize it among our different competing daily roles and goals. Many of us need more immediately noticeable reasons for being active, concrete ways we and our lives benefit every day to motivate the consistent movement that undergirds long-term sustainability.

Yes, but what if your decision to start exercising really *is* due to a health mandate? It turns out that even under those circumstances we can still find our way to our Right Why. Fortunately, creating the Right Why won't undermine your ultimate health goals. In fact, it will support them, as shown by this great personal story from renowned researcher Dan Ariely.[4]

Reward Substitution Is a Very Strategic Move

Ariely, author of *Predictably Irrational: The Hidden Forces That Shape Our Decisions* and a leading behavioral economist, discovered as a young doctoral student that he had hepatitis C. The best treatment for the condition at the time required frequent shots of interferon, which Ariely had to administer himself at home and which caused awful side effects, including extreme nausea and vomiting for sixteen hours after each injection. He resisted taking the interferon because of its side effects.

Ariely quickly realized that he wasn't motivated to give himself the shots for two reasons. First, the side effects were so unpleasant. Second, the reason for the shots was to avoid cirrhosis of the liver—an illness that wouldn't occur for another thirty years, an unimaginably far-off future.

Ariely cleverly decided to use *reward substitution* as a motivating Strategy to take the shots. He replaced a future reward (not developing cirrhosis of the liver in the far future) with a reward he could immediately experience: He would let himself watch movie marathons on the days he gave himself shots. (Since he was a doctoral student, he had this flexibility.) Once he substituted the reward of "avoid severe health consequences in thirty years" with a more immediate reward of "watch my favorite movies all day today," it was no longer as challenging to stay motivated to give himself the shots he needed. Reward substitution turned him into the most compliant patient his physicians had ever seen.

The great news is anyone can use reward substitution for any type of behavior. And the heart of Ariely's strategic solution is closely related to how you can transform physical activity from a chore you dread into a gift you can't wait to give yourself. By replacing the Wrong Why with your Right Why, you can immediately start to transform the Meaning of exercise or any self-care behavior from a chore into a gift.[5]

The Successful Cycle of Motivation

Now here's the part you may think is too easy to be true: When we change our primary reason for moving to a reason that is deeply compelling and relevant to our daily lives (that is, the Right Whys), and we also start moving in ways that feel good, our *Meaning* for exercise and physical activity effortlessly changes from negative to positive—from a chore to a gift. This transforms our perceptions and feelings about moving our bodies. Now we are motivated to move because it's something we are explicitly giving to ourselves. Let me repeat this because it's really important: *Changing your personal Meaning of exercise and physical activity from a chore into a gift will transform your relationship with movement.* (Figure 6-1 is a graphic representation that will help you remember this.)

FIGURE 6-1. From a chore to a gift.

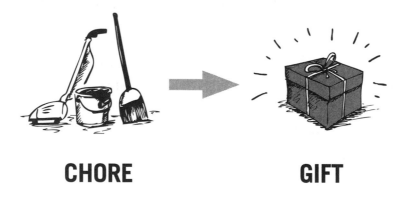

CHORE   GIFT

This radical conversion begins with a sudden, small insight but leads into a cascade that changes everything. As you find your Right Why and begin to connect with what your body really needs and wants, your Meaning of exercise shifts from a chore to a gift. Thus, instead of feeling compelled to exercise to fulfill a narrowly focused goal (such as losing twenty pounds or increasing your HDL cholesterol), you find yourself wanting to engage in movement because what you are doing makes you feel *good*. When that happens, you've escaped the Vicious Cycle of Failure and entered a much more satisfying cycle: the Successful Cycle of Motivation (Figure 6-2).

FIGURE 6-2. The Successful Cycle of Motivation.

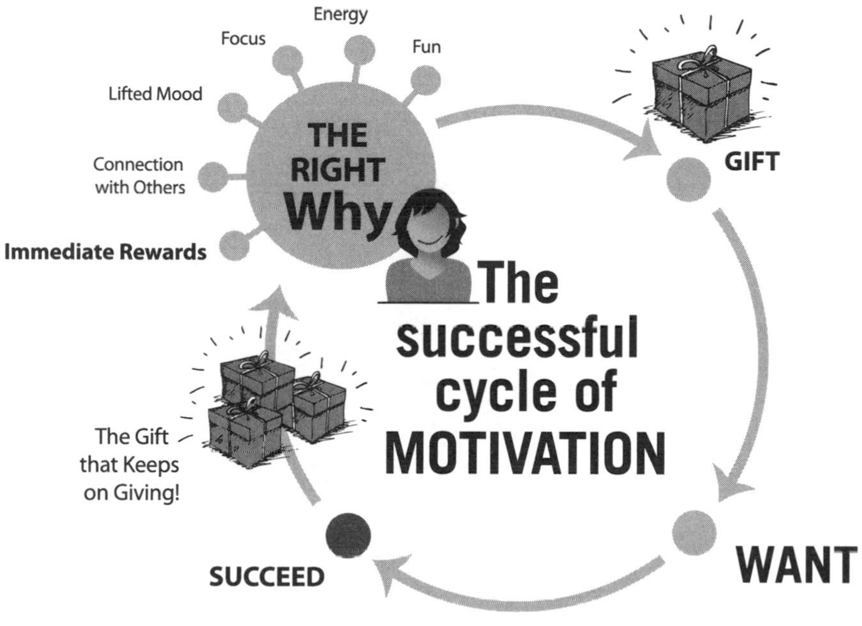

The Successful Cycle of Motivation starts from the "Right Why"—*your* Right Why. Now you are choosing to move for more relevant and compelling reasons and also choosing physical activities that give you *immediate* positive feedback: Walking for ten minutes gives you more energy, you're enjoying being in the present moment when you swim, gardening makes you smile, you're sharing stories and laughter with your close friend as you work out. Physical activity feels like a gift. Instead of a chore it's now a want because you reap rewards like fun with your family, focus at work, and feeling centered. It's the gift that keeps on giving. And you don't want it to stop.

You find that you can repeat these experiences any time you like, and this motivation becomes self-perpetuating. You feel better because you are moving your body in ways that you determine for yourself, and you naturally want to keep moving.

Listen to Your Body's Messages and Do What You Like

When I spoke to my client Cheryl about listening more to her body's messages, she wasn't sure what I meant. "Try this," I suggested. "The next time you find yourself resisting exercise or you don't want to do the workout you had planned, just stop a minute. Don't do anything. Just stop, close your eyes, and ask yourself what type of movement would feel good to do. If it's nothing, that's okay, too."

The following week, Cheryl reported back. "That was so weird," she said. "I was sitting there thinking this was a silly thing to do, and I suddenly thought—*yoga*. I wanted to do yoga, of all things. Does that even count?"

"Yoga is fine," I said, "especially if you enjoy doing it."

"Good, because I got happy just thinking about it and then I went to a class. It was fantastic."

"What do you like about it?" I asked.

"Well, I can just relax. I don't have to think about anything. We stand, we sit, we twist, sometimes we move between poses . . . Mostly we just breathe, and at the end we stretch out on the floor in *sivasana*—corpse pose—actively doing nothing." She laughed again. "That sounds even less like exercise than I thought."

"Don't worry about it. The goal is to reconnect with your preferences and likes. What you choose to do right now is not that relevant," I said. "Your body is just letting you know what it wants, and apparently this is the way it needs to move right now. Listen, and let me know what happens."

This was a good first step. Cheryl became interested in the different poses, paying attention to how each made her body feel. She moved from doing the relaxing yoga she had started with to a more athletic and flowing type of yoga experience   standing on her head, balancing with her elbows on her knees, balancing on one foot. To her surprise, she found that she was actually building muscle, strength, and flexibility from "just" doing yoga. And although she hadn't lost any weight, she told me she felt better about her body and herself. Cheryl began making time for yoga at home and going to classes on a regular basis. Because her Right Why for yoga delivered immediate gifts of well-being that she liked, she wanted to keep it up, and she had fully entered the Successful Cycle of Motivation.

Now that you understand how the Successful Cycle of Motivation works, let's check out the neuroscience that supports its premise: When we like how we feel during physical activity, we'll want to keep doing it, again and again and again.

Wanting and Liking: The Neuroscience of Reward

I love walking, my husband starts almost every day biking in our basement, one of my friends loves to ski, and my son loves to spin around until he drops. The specific physical activity people like is always going to be unique to them and often related to the moment or time of day. The key is to discover which physical activities we like doing, because our brains are set up to keep us wanting it again and again.

Research on the neuroscience of reward (the mechanisms in our brain that drive us to seek pleasurable experiences) explains why we are more motivated to pursue physical movement if it's pleasurable and helps us feel good. The neuroscience of reward is rooted in two different systems: "liking" and "wanting."[6] (It already sounds good, doesn't it?) Liking refers to the hedonic experiences that indicate states of positive feeling, such as pleasure. Wanting refers to desiring an important reward or action, something that motivates us to approach it.

According to leading neuroscientist Kent Berridge, "liking" a specific behavior (after learning that it is associated with a positive reward, like more energy) triggers "wanting" to perform that action (similar to a Pavlovian conditioned response) and consistently motivates that behavior. In addition, positive feelings actually motivate our behavior outside of our consciousness, without our even realizing this is happening.[7] This science underscores that for sustaining a physically active life, choosing to move for pleasure and other positive experiences is clearly more strategic than forcing ourselves to move in ways we don't like. It turns physical activity into something we "like" to do and will continue "wanting" to do without having to think about it.

IT'S YOUR MOVE
Moving to Feel Good

Developing your Awareness of how you really feel versus how you think you should feel and learning to act on that genuine feeling in the moment puts you in charge of decisions that you've probably been making out of habit for many years. Take a moment now to reflect on your best possible movement choices and the rewards you can reap:

» When I envision myself in an enjoyable physical activity, I see myself doing: _____

_____

» If I could choose to do any physical activity, I would choose: _____

_____

» I am at my best when I get the following experiences from physical activity: _____

_____

» I am at my worst when I get the following experiences from physical activity:_____

_____

» As a result of being active, every day I want to feel/ experience the following things: _____

_____

Now that you have more Awareness of the benefits of moving in ways you like and what feels good to you, start choosing to move in these ways and start to notice what happens.

Men and Women Might Benefit from Different Experiences

One of my primary interests as a behavioral sustainability researcher and coach has been to understand gender differences and how to best promote self-care behaviors like physical movement to both women and men. We live in a culture that bombards us with the importance of being healthy and controlling our weight, but there's been little research to see whether these messages impact men and women in the same way.

The research into high-intensity versus lower-intensity exercise that we discussed in Chapter 4 supports what we already know: What feels good is inherently subjective. Traditional exercise recommendations have been objective, one-size-fits-all prescriptions based on research linking a specific physical activity "dose" to health biomarkers and illness prevalence. But as exercise psychologist Panteleimon Ekkekakis discusses,[8] there is growing realization among leading organizations such as the American College of Sports Medicine that the intensity at which we exercise influences our feelings and whether or not we stick to it.

Some interesting population-level research conducted in Belgium suggests that there might also be gender differences between the psychological benefits we get from differing intensities of physical activity.[9] This study collected data on 6,803 adults between the ages of twenty-five and sixty-four. It found that women and men experienced mental health benefits at distinctly different intensity levels of physical activity. In men, high-intensity activity was associated with lower depression and anxiety. In women, lower-intensity activity (such as walking) was associated with enhanced emotional well-being. Regardless of whether these findings resonate with you personally, the key is to understand what type of physical movement will give you experiences that enhance how you feel immediately. Remember, it's the immediate rewards that are going to motivate you to be physically active day after day.

IT'S YOUR MOVE

Which Intensity Best Boosts Your Mood?

For physical movement to be sustainable, it's important to find activities that are right for you. In general, do you feel better when you do lower-level movement, like walking, or higher-intensity movement, like running or spinning? Or does it depend on the day?

"Gift" Yourself with Movement
Any and Every Way You Can

An important step toward embracing movement in your life is simply becoming mindful that your choices about how you move through your day truly are *your choices*. Remember, there is an infinite amount of movement available to you every day, from more structured exercise of longer durations to the many opportunities to move (OTMs). Be strategic and give yourself the gift of whatever type of movement will most benefit you and which you can fit in on any given day.

Once you start to discover activities that work and feel good, give them to yourself as gifts. Choosing to move in ways we enjoy can also liberate a love for activities that we haven't thought about in years (e.g., ice skating, bike riding, skateboarding, sledding, Hula-Hooping) or lead us to consider doing things we've never done (Pilates, salsa dancing, rock climbing, kayaking, taiko drumming). For shorter OTMs, turn on some music and dance in your living room for five minutes. If you have a letter to mail, walk to the mailbox two blocks away. Reframe housework and yard work as OTMs for your body: Dance while you sweep, carry laundry up the stairs, pull some weeds, take out the garbage. Take five to ten minutes anytime to clear your mind, run an errand, and get blood flowing throughout your body, especially your brain!

You can also expand the number of gifts you give yourself by opening up the possibilities of whom you can include. Being active is a wonderful way to spend quality time with the people or pets you love and enjoy being with. So walk with and chase your children, stroll with your partner or your whole family after dinner, walk and talk with friends. Consider having a Walking Meeting during work (as discussed in Chapter 5). But if you really want to discover the numerous gifts of movement that you could be giving yourself, read on.

Let the Games Begin!: Discovering the Gifts of Movement in Your Life

A number of my clients enjoy making a treasure hunt out of discovering gifts of movement in their daily lives. Some give themselves points for every new activity they find, while others just enjoy the process. The game of finding these hidden OTMs fosters a learning mindset that opens up more and more possibilities and makes it much easier to contend with the challenges to your plans that arise.

Inspired by my clients' experiences and enthusiasm, I created the *It's Your Move!* game board, shown in Figure 6-3. The subtitle of the game is "Give Yourself the Gift of Movement," which is the goal of the game. The game board reflects one day in your life. The game begins each morning and ends at bedtime. Your challenge is to discover and claim as many OTMs as you can each day. You make up the rules as you go along, and you can't lose—in fact, you can win many times over, every day, as you discover and claim your OTMs.

FIGURE 6-3. *It's Your Move!* game board.

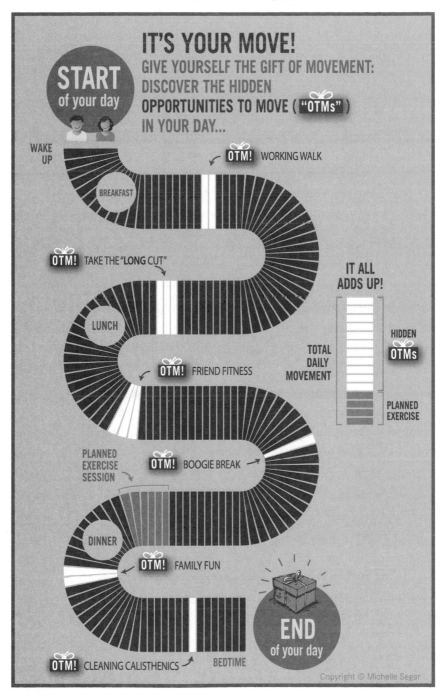

As you can see, the spaces on the board are shaded in slightly different ways. The gray spaces reflect the planned exercise session that you might already do—running, walking the dog, walking around the grocery store while you do your shopping, walking from the train to your office, and so on. It's important that you give yourself a shout-out for these wins because they too count. The white spaces represent any opportunity to move that exists—anywhere. These are examples of hidden but *potential* OTMs that you haven't noticed before now or haven't chosen to claim. Consider them as free gifts—Boogie Breaks, Working Walks, Long Cuts, Cleaning Calisthenics, and Family Fun.

We score every time we take these free gifts during the day. Note that these OTMs are not glamorous, nor do they necessitate paying for parking, changing our clothes, taking a shower, and so on. Instead, they are as mundane as can be: walking two blocks to the mailbox instead of putting the mail outside your house, for example, or going up the stairs two extra times to get more movement. If you look at the right of the game board, you see the movement counter showing the total from taking all of those extra steps. You score every time you claim an OTM, as well as every time you do a planned exercise session.

Let me give you an example of something I frequently do to claim an OTM gift in my own life. Parking is expensive on the University of Michigan campus and downtown in Ann Arbor, besides being hard to find. When I am going to a meeting or anywhere in town, I give myself ten to fifteen extra minutes to park in a surrounding neighborhood. There are multiple benefits from this one thing. I don't have to pay for parking, and I have twenty or thirty minutes to walk to and from my car, plus the energy and joy I get from moving my body outside. Is leaving early easy? No. Do I need to look at a weather report and perhaps carry an umbrella or shoes that can get wet? Yes. But the rewards I get from this Strategy motivate me to keep doing it.

Discover where and when during the space of every day you can enjoy the immediate rewards of energy and lifted mood brought by moving more throughout the day. When any and all physical activity counts, incorporating extra physical movement into daily life becomes much more realistic and possible. It makes us *want* to do more, and it also gets us curious about where and how much we can discover so that we *can* do more movement every day.

As you start becoming aware of the many OTMs you can actually give yourself during any given day, especially the kinds of physical activities that give you pleasure or feel good, you will make some interesting, unexpected, and life-changing discoveries.

Could Walking Be Your Way?

If only one physical activity could be a gift for most people, I would have to pick walking—an easy, very pleasurable, and almost always available option. Walking—not power walking and not trekking across the country, just plain old walking around the block, in your neighborhood, to the store, in the park, or through a city—is among the very best ways to sustain a physically active life. In fact, I'm not the only one on the walking bandwagon. There are organizations like America Walks and exciting national-level initiatives happening to promote walking, such as Every Body Walk![10] and the U.S. Surgeon General's first-ever national Walking Call-to-Action, scheduled to be released in 2015.[11]

Here are just a handful of reasons why walking is wonderful:

>> Walking is something most of us naturally have access to multiple times a day. We don't have to go out of our way to find it.

>> Walking lends itself to quality time with our kids and families and connecting with friends.

>> Walking feels great once we get rid of rules about how we should be doing it.

>> Walking helps us clear our minds. (It's a great way to grab some "me time.")

» Walking does double-duty as a great time to be on our own or to enjoy the company of other people.

» It can be done almost anywhere, at almost any time, and in virtually any weather.

» It can be done at any age.

» Except for a pair of good shoes, it won't cost anything.

» When we walk somewhere, anywhere, or as part of our work, it also counts as daily activity.

» It benefits our well-being and health in many ways.[12]

» Walking does all of these things, plus it "counts" as a valid form of exercise!

Walking is a perfect physical activity for so many, yet walking for exercise still strikes many people as "cheating." In fact, in the twenty years that I've been coaching people, I can honestly say that few have started our work with the belief that walking counts as valid physical activity.

But guess what? Research shows that there isn't even a difference in the amount of calories we burn between training on an elliptical and walking if we do it for the same amount of time and at the same intensity level.[13] Once people get used to the simple idea that walking counts (and it counts big time), they get excited. Why drag yourself to the gym if you'd much rather be taking a walk in the park with your family? Walking has been my main form of daily movement for the last ten years, and I love it.

When you decide you want to try walking, do it in ways that feel good to you. The neuroscience of reward does not just suggest that when we walk for pleasure, we'll like it and keep wanting to do it. Other research also shows that when people are asked to walk at a pace that maintains positive feelings, they still select intensities that have the potential to improve physiological fitness and health.[14] As Gretchen Rubin, author of *The Happiness Project*, put it: "A twenty-minute walk that I do is better than the four-mile run that I don't do."[15] Amen, sister!

Throughout the sections in this book on Meaning and Awareness, you've had an opportunity to dive into the Meanings you've had for exercise and physical activity before reading *No Sweat*, how they came to be, and the relevant science. You also had a chance to "exorcise exercise" along with other activities to help you begin the process of transforming exercise from a chore into a gift. In Chapter 7, we begin our exploration of Permission. That chapter, and Chapter 8, are the culmination of everything you've learned so far in the sections on Meaning and Awareness, but they will also generate more momentum—showing you how to truly align who you are and what you most want and need with your physical movement choices, and moving forward on your path of sustained self-care and success.

The Takeaways

- Reframing your Why from a Wrong Why (for example, a future abstract goal to be healthy) to a Right Why (for example, because it will help you achieve something tangible that you want to experience and/or find personally compelling today) transforms your motivation. The Successful Cycle of Motivation starts from the Right Why.

- "To be healthy" tends to be a Wrong Why for many people because it is too abstract and doesn't provide the immediate feedback we need to keep striving toward it. People are more motivated by immediate results than future rewards.

- There are many incredible ways that being physically active can enhance your life every day—too many to list in this book. (Just a few are improved energy, less stress, higher life satisfaction, better mood, and improved immunity.)

- Pick the Right Why that feels most compelling to you now and test-drive it for a while by selecting the physical activity that delivers it.

- Reward substitution—replacing a future reward with something positive that you can experience immediately—converts behavior from a chore into a gift you want to give yourself.

- Changing your personal Meaning of exercise and physical activity from a chore into a gift transforms your motivation and relationship with movement.

- Research in the neuroscience of reward explains why people are more motivated to pursue physical movement if it's pleasurable. Choosing to move for positive experiences is strategic for sustaining a physically active life because it turns physical activity into something you "like" to do and will continue "wanting" to do.

- Walking is a gift that virtually everyone can give themselves: It is easy, pleasurable, always available, and filled with social, soulful, and well-being benefits.

PART III

• • • • •

PERMISSION

Giving yourself PERMISSION to prioritize your own
self-care—to feel better every day—provides the fuel
for your daily roles and goals and powers
your sense of well-being.

CHAPTER

7

Permission to Prioritize Self-Care

"YOU LIED TO ME!" MINA WAS ANGRY. I WAS SO TAKEN ABACK BY HER outburst that I was momentarily at a loss for words.

It was mid-program, and we had just gotten into the topic of Permission: reflecting on what Mina had learned to prioritize in her life, where she automatically put her attention each day, and how that might be keeping her from putting self-care at the top of her to-do list. I knew that Mina had a lot on her plate. She was in a bad relationship, she was struggling to keep her small gift shop afloat, and she was painfully aware that she was letting her employees ruin her business. She was not taking charge of anything, including her own weight and health, which was her impetus to work with me.

"You lied to me," Mina repeated. "This is not about exercise. It's about my *life*!"

I thought for a moment. "You're right," I said. "When we talk about finding activities that truly give us pleasure, and the difficulty of finding time for them amid all of the other things we need to do, it's not about the exercise per se. We're really talking about why we find it so hard to make time to take care of *ourselves*."

Mina sighed deeply as her anger slowly left her body and her eyes brimmed with tears. "Okay, okay," she said, "it feels like such an insurmountable task, Michelle. Where do I start?"

So much of what we have learned over the years about taking care of ourselves boils down to simply adding a health behavior to our lives in prescribed doses: Eat five servings of fruits and vegetables, get eight hours sleep, do thirty minutes of exercise five days per week. It sounds simple, yet we are continually caught by surprise when we fail to follow through.

When taking care of ourselves is just another thing to do, it becomes a chore, one of a thousand choices that compete for our time and attention. It easily loses out to the needs of the people and things we care most about—a list on which we tend to put ourselves last. This leads to a disturbing paradox: When we do not prioritize our own self-care because we are busy serving others, our energy is not replenished. Instead, we are exhausted, and our ability to be there for anyone or anything else is compromised.

You may not even have thought about where you actually rank self-care in your list of daily tasks, but wherever it lies is probably less the result of a conscious decision than it is an unconscious product of how you were socialized—educated by your parents, the media, and your workplace expectations about the acceptable and most worthy ways to spend your time. If you think about it for even a few moments, you'll realize that if self-care truly was valued by society at large, we wouldn't even have to discuss it.

Making self-care a top daily priority may sound like a small thing and even an unnecessary thing to do. Yet I have found that deliberately giving ourselves Permission to prioritize our own self-care is an essential step to take and the key to sustaining a self-care behavior like physical activity. In fact, in my coaching, I've found that *not* giving ourselves Permission to prioritize our own self-care is what most derails our ability to sustain it, even more so than low motivation.

Does Your Mindset Have Your Best Interests in Mind?

We all have a roster of fixed *should* items on our mental to-do list—obligations and interests that we automatically believe must be taken care of. Just as our Meanings of exercise developed out of our past experiences and understandings, we have also developed a general sense about taking care of ourselves. Is it selfish or smart? Do we consider self-care optional or essential?

To successfully integrate self-care into your daily life, you need to create space in that seemingly immovable mindset for the new belief that self-care is *essential*. This is similar to having to make changes in your thinking about exercise as you did in the chapters on Meaning and Awareness. The first step is to get inside your mindset and surface the beliefs and attitudes that are preventing you from prioritizing your daily energy level and sense of well-being.

It's easy to mistake our mindset for our self and to mistake our mindset's choices for our choices. That's because our mindset is powerful. It determines how we perceive *everything*, guiding our behavior and creating our priorities for how we spend our time. Because we live inside it, seeing the world through its window, it's hard to even see. The thing to remember is this: Your mindset is your socialization, but it is not necessarily *you*. And it does not always have your best interests at heart.

Say you're hard at work, close to exhaustion from the hours you've put into a project over the last few days. You look out the window to see a beautiful day and think how refreshing it would feel to just get out there and walk around for forty-five minutes. And then you think,

No, I should finish my work first. You do finish your work, but by then it's getting dark out, and it's all you can do to drag yourself home and into bed.

Which actor in this drama is your mindset? Which is you? Which seems to have your best interests at heart?

What we value most in life is strongly influenced by socially constructed norms and pressures—needing to be "a good provider" or "a good parent." Few would argue that these are not good social values. But because they are so cherished in society, and we also get rewarded for choosing to fulfill these values, they can easily grow out of proportion. They become *shoulds* that we fulfill automatically and to excess, crowding out everything else.

When you try to add one more *should—I should take care of my own daily health and fitness*—it takes its place at the end of a long line. Once there, it faces another challenge, a really powerful social *should* that's hard for most people to get past: *I should not be selfish.* This kind of thinking, which is all wrapped up in our own values and self-worth, easily distracts us and effortlessly derails self-care.

This fixed mindset is well intentioned but misdirected. When we continually let the endless *should* tasks of our lives take priority over our own self-care needs, we feel overwhelmed, exhausted, and fatalistic about the possibility of ever changing anything. Just as we can inflame any muscle through overwork, we can also overuse our emotional-mental-physical "caretaker muscle." I call this painful state of being *caretakeritis*. Ouch!

Caretakeritis Is Not Good for Anyone's Health

Research supports what most of us know to be true in our own lives: We have real difficulty prioritizing self-care among our many other competing daily goals.[1] Caring for others and working with passion and dedication are wonderful impulses and contribute toward what makes life meaningful. But when caring for others overshadows our own daily needs and quality of life, we've lost the balance we need to

IT'S YOUR MOVE
Do You Have Symptoms of Caretakeritis?

Check the symptoms of caretakeritis that resonate with your own experience:

❑ Having difficulty saying no

❑ Responding to requests automatically, without reflecting on your own time, energy, and goals

❑ Not having your self-care and a sense of well-being as top daily priorities

❑ Consistently prioritizing your to-do list and the needs of your loved ones over your own needs, sense of well-being, and self-care

❑ Not delegating tasks to others because no one does them as perfectly as you

❑ Frequently feeling emotionally and physically exhausted as you try to keep up on the to-do treadmill, and feeling like you can't step off

❑ Feeling like you have no control to change things

generate our own energy and well-being—the literal fuel for what matters most.*

---

* Note that people who are unemployed and struggling to make ends meet have to see to their basic needs, like finding work, putting food on the table, and taking care of children. These things understandably take priority over self-care. It's important to acknowledge the very real challenges to self-care that people who are living in extreme circumstances—such as caring for newborn infants or working two or three jobs to pay their bills—have.

There are some real differences between men and women when it comes to many issues related to self-care, health status, and well-being.[2] But when some people hear me speak about caretakeritis, they assume it refers only to women who sacrifice their own needs to take care of their loved ones. Although the term seems gendered, it's not. It refers to anyone who *always* puts "taking care of business" (whatever that business is) ahead of his or her own self-care.

Although caretakeritis does not discriminate according to gender, men and women do seem to tell themselves different stories about self-care. It's common, for example, to hear women say that they fear they are being selfish when they prioritize their own self-care. When I work with men, on the other hand, I find that being selfish isn't their concern. Rather, there is something about making time for self-care that feels unmasculine to them. In general, men are far less likely to get care for themselves, whether it's going to the doctor or getting help for mental health concerns,[3] opting for silence around emotional issues.

In his book *Invisible Men*, research psychologist and author Michael E. Addis writes that "a man's masculinity is measured in large part by his ability to make his public accomplishments widely *seen* and *heard*, while keeping his inner life *silent* and *invisible*." This creates a wide range of problems, he explains, including "lower levels of health-promoting behaviors, higher levels of health risk behaviors, and higher levels of drug and alcohol abuse."[4]

The causes and symptoms can be different for men and women, but the low prioritization of self-care is pandemic. So, while men and women might avoid their own self-care for different reasons, they both feel uncomfortable making it a top priority. My client Aziz's story is typical of what happens to so many men. When Aziz first consulted me, he was at his wit's end. He had several competing roles: He was a husband, a father, part of a large extended family for which he felt responsibility, and an employee at a large financial institution. He wanted to exercise regularly, but he had an ingrained belief that it was important, above all, to be "a good provider," which meant always being available for work, including sleeping with his smartphone next to his bed. Connected to this, he had other beliefs instructing him to also be "a good son, a good husband, and a good dad," which meant that he must dedicate his time outside of work to his own parents and to his wife and children, instead of spending it on himself.

Recently, Aziz had been feeling exhausted, mildly depressed, and "out of shape." His doctor told him that he needed to work out more and eat better. Aziz wanted to comply, but he had no idea how he could accomplish any of this and still fulfill his obligations. "I certainly can't afford to lose my job," he told me. "Anyway, when I look at the other guys at work, they're just like me. I told my wife that's just the way life is—my father is the same. But she insisted, so here I am."

On the surface, fulfilling your responsibilities as a good son, husband, father, or employee seems to have nothing to do with exercising. Yet Aziz's belief system about his priorities as an individual, and especially as a man, generated a subtle anxiety about taking time to exercise, which undermined his ability to take better care of himself. What's really important to know is that he, like most of us, wasn't aware that any of this was going on because it's how we've been socialized to prioritize.

In fact, taking care of others and accomplishing all of the tasks on our to-do lists can actually be addictive. In the workplace, people who can't stop working are called workaholics, yet they are simultaneously admired for sticking with the company, going the extra mile, and getting the job done despite everything. We get satisfaction from our ability to take care of business and see to the needs of others, and we get gold stars from society. We're praised and rewarded by career advancement and the grateful thanks of friends and family. But if you feel driven to take care of everything or everyone else, virtually all of the time, sooner or later you are going to burn out—or worse.

Are You Paying Attention to
Your Body's Distress Signals?

Exhaustion. Anxiety. Depression. Unexplained pain. When you tune out everyday stress messages (your back hurts from sitting for hours, you're tired because you need more sleep), your body turns up the volume and starts screaming in the form of more serious physical and emotional aches and pains. While their connection to the original source may be lost, their painful effects are very much present. Ironically, while we ignore our physical distress signals, we simultaneously make it a point to stay connected to the digital world so we don't miss any electronic messages. On we go, cramming as much productivity as we can into every day, just hoping that the bucket doesn't overflow.

On the morning of April 6, 2007, Arianna Huffington, author of *Thrive* and the editor-in-chief of the Huffington Post Media Group, collapsed in her office from exhaustion and lack of sleep and hit her head on the corner of her desk, resulting in a cut eye and a broken cheekbone. Burnout, stress, and sleep deprivation are not limited to media stars, however. These are all common issues we face as humans living in the hyper-connected digital age.

It doesn't take scientific research to recognize the problem before your head hits the desk. You probably know scores of people, including yourself, who simply don't sleep enough, whether it's through choice or not. We sleep less so we can work beyond our limits or connect more; we sleep less because our minds are racing with all the things we need to get done the next day. The symptoms of burnout are probably all too familiar to you: exhaustion on a physical and emotional level, not feeling engaged or accomplished, feeling resentment toward or even detachment from your own life. You're tired, you can't concentrate, you feel angry and anxious and depressed, and you keep doing the same thing because it's likely that you don't have the energy to figure out how to change things . . . Sounds a lot like caretakeritis, doesn't it?

Because our socialization for getting healthier and preventing disease has been dominated by messages that we should focus on external outcomes like changing the numbers on a scale, we often don't notice *how we feel* during the day or even consider a behavior as essential as sleep to be a core self-care behavior we should work on.

Our global tendency to keep doing and not renewing only seems to be growing. According to the American Psychological Association's "Stress in America" study, "High stress and ineffective coping mechanisms . . . appear to be ingrained in our culture, perpetuating unhealthy lifestyles and behaviors for future generations."[5] Lack of sleep, for example, is thought to contribute to catching everyday illnesses like colds and flus, as well as increasing our risk of developing many illnesses.[6] When we don't get enough sleep, we wake up exhausted and often in a foul mood—the exact opposite of being fueled to enjoy and succeed at our most cherished roles and responsibilities.

In contrast to the expansive and creative thinking that positive emotions evoke, when we experience negative emotions, like anxiety or stress, our thinking narrows,[7] reducing our ability to make good decisions or see opportunities right in our midst. Stress promotes the thought "I can't do it. I don't have time." It seems as if people who manage to be regularly physically active *and* get things done must somehow have more time available. But of course, they don't—we all live in the same twenty-four hours. The protestation "I don't have time to be physically active" feels like the core issue. But I've learned that for many, it is a smoke screen hiding what's really going on: *not intentionally prioritizing being physically active.*

So maybe a better question is this: Why do some people prioritize fitting physical activity into their days while others don't?

Seeing Through the "I Don't Have Time" Smoke Screen

Individuals who are regularly active don't literally have more time, but they somehow make it work. Self-care is a high priority for them, and they make sure to schedule time for it. They make it a priority despite time constraints because they know that their daily quality of life and performance is enhanced when they are physically active—they simply enjoy it, or they feel that it benefits them in real ways, such as reducing their stress or helping them focus. When they're not active, they feel it. They're sluggish, tense, and unhappy.

My husband, Jeff, is a perfect example of this. He gets up every day around 5 a.m. to exercise in our basement on a stationary bike and lift weights. Because asking about motivation is my job (and because this is a time when I am fast asleep), I did just that. At first he told me it was because he wanted to "be healthy"—his late father had a history of heart disease, which he wants to avoid. I know that many people automatically answer "to be healthy" because they haven't really given it much thought and that so clearly seems the obvious answer. So I pushed further. "Okay, but is being healthy your motivator for getting up every morning when your alarm rings and you've gotten only about six hours of sleep?" (I'm allowed to say this as his wife.)

"No," he said. "It's because if I don't exercise, I feel like crap." Again, as his wife, I know this to be true.

He and I follow the gender divide found by research when it comes to the effects of not sleeping: He can get by on less sleep, while for me, sleep is my number one nutrient. If I don't get enough sleep, I feel awful. For me, sleep provides energy for the most important parts of my life, the parts that reflect who I am and what I care most about. I think of my self-care as "sustain-ergy"—a daily energizer that fuels what matters most. So sleep is the foundation of my self-care hierarchy, while exercise is Jeff's. See our distinct self-care hierarchies in Figure 7-1.

Despite our differing self-care hierarchies, my husband and I have this in common: We deeply understand that our foundational self-care behavior makes or breaks our day. And we do everything we can to help each other meet our respective daily self-care needs.

FIGURE 7-1. Jeff's and Michelle's Self-Care Hierarchies.

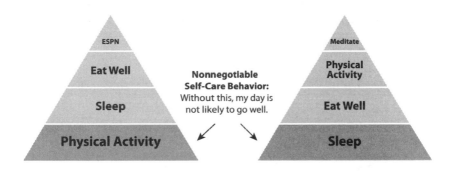

Understanding these very real consequences on feeling and functioning makes our self-care nonnegotiable. Although we still do some *shoulding* on ourselves (it's hard to break away from our socialization completely) and we both have an extreme work ethic, this does not prevent us from consistently claiming our essential self-care activity. I need sleep, he needs exercise, and we both make time to get it most of the time.

Your Daily Self-Care Needs

The many contexts in which we grow up, live, and work all teach us what to believe, which rules to obey, and which goals to value and pursue.[8] The first job of these beliefs is to get us through our first years in one piece; over time, they guide our important decisions and, ultimately, our entire life. By the time we are mature adults, our beliefs and belief systems about self-care have "mapped" our brains, forming neural connections and pathways that our thoughts follow automatically and unconsciously—creating our self-care mindset. As we will see, this mindset is not hardwired, although it certainly feels that way.

The beliefs we hold come from our socialization and interactions with living our lives.[9] They actually help form the organization of our self, our concept of who we are.[10] Learning new beliefs is so much work that sometimes it can seem impossible. Yet understanding that beliefs are indeed the foundation of our choices, and ultimately our destiny, illuminates how crucial it is to start with our beliefs when deciding to learn how to adopt any new self-care behavior. In fact, learning is the process whereby "new information leads to a change in beliefs,"[11] the necessary condition for transforming our opinions, preferences, and ultimately our ability to sustain a lifetime of fitness and self-care.

Because we learn our beliefs as children, we credit those beliefs with greater wisdom than our own small selves, and we give them the same kind of power we grant to the adults in our lives. As adults, we still obey these ingrained rules and demands. At the same time, we have the nagging feeling that some deeper, essential part of ourselves is not being nourished or heard. Our adult insights and true core needs are often shouted down by the louder voices that tell us what we should be doing instead.

Yet, it is vital to our well-being and health and to fulfilling our potential to become aware of the deep-seated and unexamined beliefs that have been directing our decisions. Likewise, it is vital to have a frank conversation with ourselves about whether or not these beliefs—which guide us to automatically prioritize our many daily tasks, responsibilities, and pleasures—are actually supporting or undermining the best interests of our core self: that voice inside that is so hard to hear over the daily chorus of *shoulds*.

The term *self-care* actually encapsulates the core issue we are talking about: *caring for* ourselves by making sure we continually replenish our energy and support our well-being. Because of our socialization, we often don't think about our well-being. In fact, *well-being* is an unappreciated term. When we use it, we often just think about feeling "positive." Yet let's consider what the word *being* actually means. *Being* is a form of the verb "be," which refers to both "existence" and "being who we are," so well-being really means that we are doing a great job of being who we are!

IT'S YOUR MOVE
Daily Self-Care Needs Assessment

Before you can give yourself Permission to get your daily self-care needs met, it's important to know what they are. Try this assessment.

1. Close your eyes for a moment and recall a time when you felt at ease, grounded in yourself, without worry. (If you can't recall such a moment, just imagine what it might be like for you.) Visualize what was going on and what you were experiencing with your senses, your emotions, your body, and your mind. This is your glimpse of well-being.

2. Now read the list below. Check the experiences you need more of to get to that place of well-being. Check as few or as many experiences as resonate with you. Write in any that may be missing.

To have a greater sense of well-being in my life, I need to feel:

❏ Less stress   ❏ Relaxed
❏ Strong   ❏ More fun
❏ In a better mood   ❏ Proud of myself
❏ Competent   ❏ Creative
❏ Powerful   ❏ Loved
❏ Centered   ❏ Engaged
❏ Inspired   ❏ Curious
❏ More meaning   ❏ More vitality
❏ Autonomous   ❏ Self-worth
❏ Less anxious   ❏ Other(s) _____
❏ Joyful

Go back and circle the two experiences you are *most* in need of having in your day now. Once you've identified the most important gap in your daily self-care needs, let's figure out what might help you fill it. Figure 7-2 is a blank My Self-Care Hierarchy. Based on the two most important daily self-care needs you identified, *which* self-care behavior do you think might be able to help you realize those two self-care needs and experiences? Is it sleep, physical activity, meditation, reading a great book, or taking a bath before bed every night? You might not know now, but you can start experimenting to find out. Take the self-care behavior you think it might be, and list it as your foundational, nonnegotiable self-care behavior at the bottom of the hierarchy. Don't worry; these hierarchies are not set in stone. They change whenever we determine that another self-care behavior is more foundational to our daily self-care needs, which also change.

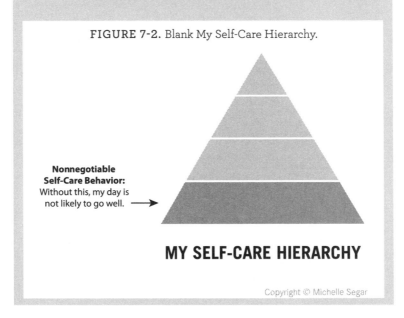

FIGURE 7-2. Blank My Self-Care Hierarchy.

Nonnegotiable Self-Care Behavior: Without this, my day is not likely to go well. ⟶

MY SELF-CARE HIERARCHY

Give Yourself Permission to Stop Following *Shoulds*

Allowing yourself to let go of the external guidance of *shoulds* can seem daunting, even scary. After all, they've accompanied you throughout your entire life. It may feel like these *shoulds* own you—and, in a way, they do, because our beliefs do determine our decisions. Yet we've been let down over and over again by the beliefs and rules about how to be healthy and take care of ourselves that we grew up with and have continued to repeat throughout our lives. (Think, for example, of achieving that "perfect" number on the bathroom scale.) But we're used to them and so we follow them effortlessly.

I've also come to believe that, on a deeper level, daily decision making and behavior based on "I should" lets us off the hook of taking personal responsibility for our own decisions, actions, or inactions. Although we think of ourselves as being responsible when we check off all of the *shoulds* on our daily lists, we're often just taking the path of least resistance. It is generally much easier in the moment to do what we feel is expected of us than it is to do the hard work of figuring out what it is *we* want to experience in our day and get out of life.

This doesn't have to be your reality, though. Instead of being guided by your *shoulds*, you can take ownership of your life, identify your daily needs, and let them guide your decisions. This will free you to refuel your energy and sense of self so you can foster what you most care about.

Make no mistake. This is a big idea to take in, especially if you feel responsible for *everything*. Let's go back to my meeting with Mina from the beginning of this chapter. When we got to this point in our conversation, Mina boiled over again. "But there *are* a million things I really should do. And I can't seem to do half of them, let alone make time to get some exercise."

"When we say *I really should do this*," I explained, "what we often mean is *I'm doing this because it's something that I think I'm supposed to do*. But when we make decisions primarily to fulfill an infinite to-do list of *shoulds*, that actually prevents us from *mindfully* evaluating each daily choice based on its merits and whether or not it helps us achieve the things that we most value and want in our lives. And this takes us farther away from ourselves and our potential. In fact, we can't really experience well-being if we're driven to fulfill what we think we should while also ignoring what *we* need and want." I paused to make sure she was taking this in.

"Look, Mina," I continued, "I won't kid you: Assuming autonomy and responsibility for your own self-care is a big, big deal. A lot of things will change. You have to actively go after it—no one is going to hand it to you. Simply *wishing you could* incorporate self-care into your life is not enough. You have to decide that it is *essential* for you. In my experience, believing that self-care is essential and a real priority is the hardest part."

She frowned. "Believing it?" Mina pondered this for a moment. "I guess I actually don't believe it. I can't even imagine believing it."

"What *do* you believe about getting active and taking better care of yourself?"

She shrugged. "I've never given it much thought. I just know I'm supposed to do it. For my health and weight, etc." Mina sounded so discouraged, like she'd just come up against a brick wall, with no way to get through it.

"Would you try a thought experiment for me?" I asked.

She looked startled. "What's that?"

"It's just pretending," I replied, smiling. "No commitments."

"Sure, I guess."

"Okay. Close your eyes. Now just pretend that your mindset is giving you this message: *Mina, feeling good is your top priority today.*" Mina made a face, shifted around uncomfortably, and finally settled down. I let her breathe for a moment. "How do you feel about that idea?"

She didn't look happy or like she knew what to do. She shrugged, eyes still closed.

"Remember, Mina, we're just pretending ."

With that reminder, Mina seemed to relax. She smiled and just sat for a while. "I'm starting to feel the tension go out of my shoulders."

"What do you pretend to believe about time for your self-care and feeling good right now?"

"I pretend for this moment to believe that doing something small every day to take better care of myself will help. Also, I'm feeling curious, wondering whether I could take ten minutes to just go outside and breathe some fresh air or even leave work early so I can take a bath before going to sleep."

"And how does that idea make you feel?"

"Lighter. Happy. Proud of myself." She opened her eyes, startled. "Whoa!"

Mina's resistance to change is a wall I frequently face with clients. Framing the new ideas as pretending or just an experiment frees people up to give it a try, just as Mina did.

IT'S YOUR MOVE
Pretend

Try the simple thought experiment that I asked Mina to do. Imagine that you have a new mindset that is directing you to make feeling better in your daily life and self-care a *top priority*. Consider one or two small things that you could give yourself Permission to do in your day that would recharge your battery and bring positive feelings:

1. What activities would you spend time doing?

2. When you imagine yourself doing these activities, what do you notice or feel about yourself?

Your Brain Can Change, and So Can Your Mindset

Changing your mindset takes longer than one simple thought exercise, but it is possible to do. The adult brain, contrary to what you may believe, is not irrevocably set in its way of thinking. "The brain," writes Norman Doidge in *The Brain That Changes Itself*, "can change its own structure and function through thought and activity."[12] This fascinating phenomenon is called neuroplasticity. In a review on neuroplasticity, Richard Davidson, a pioneer in affective neuroscience, and his coauthor, Bruce McEwen, report that interventions, such as cognitive therapy and certain forms of meditation, result in structural and functional changes in the brain.[13] Research in this area suggests that programs that help us change our beliefs and the way we think about things, such as learning new MAPS to fitness and self-care, can create literal changes in our brain. Davidson and McEwen suggest that we should consider our efforts to change our thinking and feelings about things as mental training, similar to building a new skill. They conclude by noting that "just as practice will improve musical performance and produce correlated regionally specific anatomical changes,"[14] training ourselves to think differently changes our brain. This puts to rest any notion that "it's too late to change." The research clearly shows that it's not.

You *can* change a lifetime of thinking and behavior. The necessary starting place is giving yourself Permission to do so.

Permission Is the Gateway to Prioritizing Your Self-Care

We talk a lot in everyday conversation about giving ourselves consent and approval (e.g., "I gave myself permission to go to the movies yesterday"). Just saying something like that feels thrilling and somewhat illicit. Acting on it feels empowering. Aziz's experience with Permission shows how powerful reprioritizing self-care can be.

"When you mentioned caretakeritis," Aziz told me, "I thought it was just for women. I almost quit working with you right then. But when I thought about it for a while, I realized that it actually did apply to me. I had caretakeritis from putting the important needs of my family and my work before my own all of the time! For years I had the habit of using anything as an excuse not to have time to take care of myself. That realization really rocked my world. I realized that if I was going to give my family and job the best I could and enjoy doing it, I needed to make different choices."

I asked him how he began doing that. He answered:

Well, we'd talked about Permission, and I thought about what that could mean in the real world. I started by giving myself Permission to stop working forty-five minutes earlier on most days. *[He often works until 6:30 and misses dinner with his family.]* I also gave myself Permission to turn my phone off during dinner so I wouldn't be tempted to answer it if it rang.

I now say no to many things that interfere with the time I've scheduled to exercise. I found out that the world didn't stop because I got off for a few hours a week to exercise. While that realization was a blow to my ego at first, it became a relief. While I know it will take a while to see whether I'll be successful for the rest of my life, my mindset has drastically changed about taking care of myself and my health. I feel happier now, and even my kids noticed.

When we give ourselves Permission, we are acknowledging that we are *the* gatekeeper of our lives. We are taking charge as we tend to our deepest self-care needs as human beings, independent of our roles and responsibilities.

The moment we accept personal responsibility for our own quality of daily life, the radical transformation has already begun from reluctantly following future-oriented, externally motivated "health" behavior to intentionally responding to our very real self-care needs.

We can't take care of ourselves, feel our best, or thrive if we don't claim time to renew ourselves and foster our own well-being. As with any underdeveloped muscle, strengthening our "self-care muscle" can be uncomfortable to do at first. Expect it, start small, but give yourself Permission to feel the discomfort and possible anxiety that comes with changing your beliefs about such a core issue, especially when it may relate to your relationships and past patterns with others.

Bottom line: If you don't mindfully give yourself Permission to prioritize time for your own self-care, no one else will.

IT'S YOUR MOVE
How Ready Are You to Take Better Care of Yourself?

How ready do you feel to give yourself Permission to take better care of yourself? Rank your answer from 1 (not at all ready) to 10 (ready right now).

1   2   3   4   5   6   7   8   9   10
Not Ready   **Very Ready**

If You're Not Ready, Pretend You Are

We can move self-care and time for ourselves to the top of our to-do lists only if we feel genuinely comfortable making these things top priorities. Even if you don't feel this way yet, *pretend you do*. For example:

» Consciously give yourself Permission to create some time in your day today, tomorrow, or the next day to enhance your sense of well-being.

» Pick a small self-care activity that will help you realize greater well-being.

» Schedule that self-care activity in your planner or smartphone and treat it like a meeting you can't miss—just to see what this feels like and how you feel afterward.

» Talk to your friends, coworkers, and family about this idea. Ask them how they feel about it. This will help start a conversation and get others thinking about it too. Talking openly about self-care and how it influences our day helps us to become more mindful in our daily choices and to acknowledge the importance of making sure we intentionally carve out time to refuel ourselves. It might also be the impetus for creating a culture change in your social circles and workplace that more highly values self-care.

When we take time to reflect on our lives and then act to make them more in accord with our core selves, we not only transform ourselves—we can transform our world.

Starting the process of giving yourself Permission to do or not do an action makes you accountable to yourself. It forces you to acknowledge that you are the person in charge of your life. The buck stops here! Permission also gives you an opportunity to actually decide how you want to live and not just let life happen to you. It brings you to your essence and core. And that's exciting.

How about adopting a learning mindset about your self-care? Experiment with a variety of things to see what works best for you. Begin now to start to try on some different Permissions and investigate their impact on making your own well-being a top daily priority.

IT'S YOUR MOVE
Making Space for Daily Self-Care

The following three steps will get you on the road to successfully making space in your brain for a fresh way of approaching self-care.

STEP 1: DECIDE

Make the conscious decision that you want to work on taking better care of yourself. Answer the following questions:

» In general, do you have the sense of well-being and greater balance that you'd like to have in your life? *Why? / Why not?*

» What are the specific consequences you experience from not taking sufficient time for your self-care?

» Are you ready to experiment with creating space in your life for having a greater sense of well-being and quality of life? *Why? / Why not?*

» *In theory,* do you want to make self-care a higher priority in your daily life?
    a. Yes
    b. No

STEP 2: MAKE SPACE

To begin making space for a new way of thinking, you need to put names to your *shoulds*. Identify your specific entrenched beliefs that conflict with your new intended belief that prioritizing self-care behaviors every day is essential (for example, "My family should always come first"). You may encounter immediate push-back even thinking about these beliefs—which is a sign that you're in the right ballpark! But above all else, be gentle with yourself during this process and don't judge it or yourself. This is about investigating and maybe even changing some foundational parts of yourself.

List three of the beliefs that conflict with the idea that your self-care should be one of your top priorities:

Belief 1. _____.
I learned this belief from _____.

» If you have (or might have) children, would you want them to hold this same belief? *Yes / No*

» Write the number from 1 (not ready) to 10 (really ready) that best represents how *ready* you feel to actually let go of this belief now: _____.

Belief 2. _____.
I learned this belief from _____.

» If you have (or might have) children, would you want them to hold this same belief? *Yes / No*

» Write the number from 1 (not ready) to 10 (really ready) that best represents how *ready* you feel to actually let go of this belief now: _____.

Belief 3. _____.
I learned this belief from _____.

» If you have (or might have) children, would you want them to hold this same belief? **Yes / No**

» Write the number from 1 (not ready) to 10 (really ready) that best represents how *ready* you feel to actually let go of this belief now: _____.

This is a time to have compassion toward yourself. You don't have to excavate any of those entrenched beliefs if you don't feel ready. The most important thing is just to get them out into the light of day so you can start to consider their truth and value to you *now*.

STEP 3: TRY ON SOME PERMISSIONS

In this step, you can "try on" Permission, just to see how it would feel to claim time that is devoted to your self-care and to increase your sense of well-being. Remember, this is just an experiment to explore new ways of thinking!

Think about this: If you were going to make your self-care and daily well-being a priority on most days, what Permissions would you need to give yourself? (Examples are Permission to take care of yourself, to talk to your family about your self-care needs, and to try that Zumba class and leave work on time on Mondays.) Now try them on for size. (Remember, this is just an experiment. You are not committing to these things.)

» I will let myself "try on" the following three Permissions so I can better fuel myself—just to see how they feel:

1. _____

2. _____

3. _____

Write the number next to each Permission—from 1 (not at all) to 10 (very difficult)—that reflects how difficult you think it's going to be to actually adopt these specific Permissions.

At this point, you've started experimenting with the idea of giving yourself Permission to make your own daily self-care needs a priority so you can take better care of yourself. Now let's dive deeper, in Chapter 8, into how when we take better care of ourselves we not only feel better but also fuel what matters most.

The Takeaways

- Your self-care mindset (your deep-seated beliefs about your priorities and the value of self-care) can prevent you from believing that your own self-care and sense of well-being belong at the top of your priority list.

- Caretakeritis—feeling overwhelmed, exhausted, and fatalistic about the possibility of ever changing anything or having enough time—results from allowing your endless *should* tasks to take priority over your own self-care needs. Caretakeritis keeps you depleted.

- When you tune out everyday messages from your body and don't take care of yourself in basic ways like getting enough sleep, you put yourself on a path of unhappiness, low productivity, and even serious physical and emotional issues.

- Because your brain can change (neuroplasticity), you can give yourself Permission to change your self-care mindset, let go of *I should*, and take ownership of your beliefs and behavior so you can better enjoy and succeed at what matters most.

- Giving yourself Permission to prioritize your own self-care is the key to make regular physical activity a reality.

- Understand your own self-care hierarchy and what your foundational, nonnegotiable behavior is.

- If you don't take care of yourself, no one else is going to do it for you.

8

What Sustains Us, We Sustain

AN OLD CLIENT OF MINE, CHAR, HAD FIRM INTENTIONS TO BE PHYSI-cally active. She cemented them by signing up for Zumba classes at the community center and planning regular walks with a friend. But she rarely made it to either one because her family responsibilities always came first—and between the needs of her three children and her husband, she had a lot of responsibilities. "I understand that it's in my best interests to give priority to exercise," she explained, "but I'm not going to tell my five-year-old that I can't take him to the park with his friends because *I'm* going for a walk in the park with *my* friend. That's just selfish."

"Being a good wife and mother is a wonderful purpose, Char," I told her, "and putting your family's needs first is often the right thing to do. But if I understand you correctly, your family's needs *always* come first. Do you always need to choose between taking care of your family and taking care of yourself?"

"Yes, I think I do," she replied. "If it's them or me, I have to pick them."

"But is it really an either/or choice? Is it possible that those two goals—taking care of your family and taking care of yourself—can actually support each other rather than compete?"

"What do you mean?" she asked.

"Well, can you think of a way that getting your own time for physical activity might actually *help* you be a good wife and mother rather than get in your way?"

"No," she said, shaking her head.

"Take your time. Think about how you feel when you've had a really great workout or enjoyed a walk with your friend."

Char thought hard. "I might be in a better mood, which I'm sure my husband would appreciate . . . I'd probably have more energy for everybody . . . Maybe I wouldn't catch every single cold my kids bring home . . ." She smiled. "Yeah, okay. I never looked at it that way. It looks really different."

"Maybe this week you could just give some thought to the message you send when you give all your energy to them and none to yourself," I suggested. "By taking care of yourself *and* your family, you can be an important role model for them as well."

But making regular self-care a consistent priority is much more challenging than these words make it sound. We often don't make the connection between deciding not to go to an exercise class we signed up for or a planned walk with friends and feeling selfish about prioritizing our own self-care. But this hidden relationship is present in many people and sabotages self-care outside our conscious awareness.

Our brain biology makes it easy for us to continue believing the core beliefs we've internalized, despite having evidence against them.[1] Sometimes, even the deep understanding that we're hurting ourselves when we cut corners on self-care isn't enough to make us change our beliefs and priorities because it's so much easier to keep believing what we've always believed. Some of my clients have had a very hard time letting go of the moralistic view that taking time to increase their sense of well-being and help them feel "good" is hedonistic and selfish. Remember, even powerful people like Arianna Huffington have trouble giving themselves Permission. She had to collapse from exhaustion to notice that her beliefs about self-care and what constitutes success were leading her in a harmful direction. We shouldn't need a health crisis to understand and appreciate our very real biological need for revitalization and self-care. Yet, in my experience, deciding that self-care is a top daily priority and then living that decision out in daily life is *the* most challenging part of the entire MAPS process. Our ultimate success with sustainability, however, depends on making this fundamental shift.

Over the years, I have encountered all sorts of resistance to this idea, much of it intense. But it finally led me to discover a compelling way to convince men, women, and even global organizations of the real, essential value of self-care: that feeling good and the positive emotions and experiences that result from self-caring pursuits like physical activity are actually revitalizing and fuel us to achieve our most meaningful roles and goals.[2]

You Are the Energy Center of Your Life

My former client Isla, a writer, described her ongoing experience with the idea of giving herself Permission to put self-care first. Her words capture the struggles, realizations, and successes of this deceptively simple but life-changing process:

> At first, I felt uncomfortable and even a little scared by the ideas we were talking about—giving myself Permission to prioritize my own well-being. I've been hiding my head in the sand my whole life about this—over half a century!—so coming up and out and staring these issues in the face was not comfortable at all. Yet

my gut told me that if I didn't face this and do something about it, my life would remain someone else's. I had been surviving for years, but not thriving. I yearned to feel more aligned with myself. Even deeper down, I sensed that if I continued to table my own yearnings, poor health would come calling. So I felt like I'd better pay attention to this message.

I was used to feeling like I need to tend to everyone I care about, even strangers I'd run into on the street. But I'm beginning to understand that by doing that, I'm giving away all of my energy to other people and things and leaving my own tank dry.

The amazing thing I have started to realize is that by using energy and time to do the things I need to feel my best and ground myself (meditation, walking in nature), I find that I have more time and energy for everything else. I don't really get how this works, but it's truly amazing.

This is the real gift, the gift only you can both give and receive: Permission to make your own self-care needs and sense of well-being a top priority.

You are the energy center of your life, the hub of the wheel. To generate optimal momentum, you need to make sure that you have all the energy you need every day for the things that matter and the people you love. Thankfully, you can refuel daily from an infinitely renewable energy source: physical movement that lifts your spirits and provides the energy that allows you to be fully present so you can make the right choices to thrive in your busy, complex life.

The Amazing Paradox of Self-Care: Giving to Yourself Means Giving More to Others

It's common sense to think that when we give something away, we no longer have it. But as Isla discovered, the amazing paradox of self-care reveals that the opposite is true: The more energy you give to caring for yourself, the more energy you have for everything else.

"I discovered this cool positive feedback loop," Isla told me. "It's such a different experience from when I start with a *should*. Somehow the same thing, when I did it because I thought I ought to, actually detracted from my whole experience. It dragged me down. Now when I do it and I'm choosing to do it, I'm using it as my daily fuel. I feel great. It energizes me, and it actually compounds exponentially. I have more energy from noticing, and then I do everything with relish—enjoy doing it—and find myself with more positive feelings. It's exponential."

The drastic difference between what Isla experienced from her activities because she felt like she ought to and doing them because she chose to do them underscores the research on framing behaviors as work or fun, and as orders or autonomy. As self-determination theory predicts, when Isla took ownership of her choices and behavior, she not only generated higher quality motivation to keep it up—she also felt energized by her choices.

"Giving myself Permission to live intentionally," Isla explained, "out of what I most care about and want to fuel, focuses my decisions and honestly delivers what I hope for on most days. And accepting the down days—instead of hating them—has also drastically increased my quality of life. I wish it wouldn't have taken me fifty-three years to learn this important thing, but I feel grateful that I have discovered this and can live my next fifty years with this new mindset."

Alchemy: The Gift of Physical Movement Becomes Essential Fuel for What Matters Most

The old phrase "energy in, energy out" traditionally refers to the balance between the energy you put into your body through eating (energy in) and the energy you put out through exercising (energy out). This is the world my exercise physiologist husband lives in. But in my motivation paradigm, "energy in, energy out" means that when we revitalize and refuel ourselves with physical movement and other self-care activities (energy in), we have that much more energy with which to care about, care for, and be with others and to create our best life (energy out).

Permission is powerful, moving us into a deeper engagement with our lives by tending to our own needs and aspirations through self-care behaviors like physical activity. This process is like alchemy, a medieval practice that tried to turn ordinary metal into gold. When we consciously choose to move to revitalize ourselves, we transform physical movement into much more than just a gift of positive rewards and feelings. We convert it into a specific vehicle for fueling ourselves on all levels—biological, emotional, and even spiritual—as we affirm ourselves and our lives. Physical activity becomes much more than just the gift of a walk in the park or a workout at the gym. We previously transformed physical movement from a chore to a gift; now we are alchemists, transmuting this gift into our essential fuel for what matters most in our lives (see Figure 8-1).

FIGURE 8-1. From a gift to essential fuel.

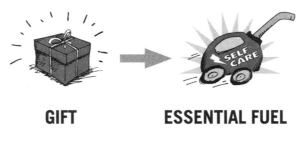

GIFT   **ESSENTIAL FUEL**

This new transformation changes *everything*. We began with a process targeting motivation, creating a new Meaning for and positive association with physical activity. Now we are focusing on our priorities, putting physical activity at the top of the list, so it can power the rest of our lives. Our beliefs about self-care also undergo an alchemical transformation. What may have seemed self-centered or even selfish can now be seen for what it is: very, very strategic.

IT'S YOUR MOVE
Wholeness, Health, and Well-Being

The English word *health* is said to be derived from the Old English *hale,* meaning "wholeness, being whole, sound or well." *Hale,* in turn, comes from the Proto-Indo-European root *kailo,* meaning "whole, uninjured, of good omen."[3] Reflect on these questions:

» When do you feel whole and centered? Be specific.

» Are there ways you move your body, or could move your body, that help you feel whole and centered?

» Are there places in which you move your body, or could move your body, that help you feel whole and centered?

» Are there people who help you feel whole and centered? Would you consider inviting them to do physical activities with you?

The understanding that self-care is a practical tool that we can use to fuel our daily functioning and performance changes the essential nature of self-care and its role in our lives. In this new mindset, self-care is no longer a goal competing with other daily responsibilities. Instead, it's the power source, an autonomous facilitator of everything we want to accomplish. That's huge! This new role for self-care transforms our self-care activities (such as daily movement, enough sleep, a balanced diet, and time for ourselves) from a gift, a powerful reward, into a personally meaningful act.

Self-care through physical activity helps us with being fully who we are—*being* a patient parent, *being* an engaged professional, *being* a loving partner, *being* a creative individual—converting every opportunity we take to move into something essential. When your daily actions and choices grow out of doing what matters most to you, you are *being* yourself really well.

You have *well-being*.

The Sustainable Cycle of Self-Care

"If you ask me why [I exercise]," *New York Times* columnist Jane Brody wrote, "weight control may be my first answer, followed by a desire to live long and well." As I read her words, I felt nervous. This comment reflected her recent interview with me about my research on how to motivate sustainable physical activity, and I had no idea what she was going to say. Her comment did not seem to bode well about her very public commentary on my perspective. As I read her next words, however, I relaxed: "But that's not what gets me out of bed before dawn to join friends on a morning walk . . . It's how these activities make me feel: more energized, less stressed, more productive, more engaged and, yes, happier—better able to smell the roses and cope with the inevitable frustrations of daily life."[4]

I let out a deep breath and smiled.

Brody's real-life realization wonderfully illustrates the many dimensions of and links between movement, motivation, self-care, and well-being that we have talked about in this book. It also illustrates the deep disconnect between how we've been socialized to think of exercise and what is actually going to motivate us to stick with it:

> » She recognized that her explicit reasons to exercise (the ones she'd tell you if you asked) were tied to how she'd been social-

ized to exercise, specifically its value in fostering health, longevity, and weight control.

» But when she dug deeper into what has actually driven her consistent years of exercising, she realized that the decision to not press the snooze button but to get out of bed and exercise every morning was motivated by how physical activity makes her feel, rather than its logical health-promoting function.

» And she went further: Brody also articulated that she was motivated to stick with exercise because it enabled her to better enjoy living and be resilient in the face of challenges.

Brody's insights offer a perfect window into the importance of radically changing our mindset about self-care behaviors like exercise, changing our Meanings for them, changing our Awareness of their very real benefits for our daily lives, and giving ourselves Permission to bring them to the front of the line as we decide what's most important every day.

Upon reflection, Brody noticed that her early-morning exercise energized her and enabled her to cope with daily frustrations. She hadn't consciously realized these benefits until she gave it thought. But once she did, she was able to recognize the powerful role physical activity had in her life because of its impressive influence on her daily feeling and functioning. Once we start understanding the very real links between how movement helps us be who we are and live our best life, we want to create them again and again.

The Sustainable Cycle of Self-Care (shown in Figure 8-2) starts in a very different place than the Vicious Cycle of Failure (Figure 2-1) and even the Successful Cycle of Motivation (Figure 6-2). In this third and final cycle, we are no longer motivated by a Wrong Why or the Right Why. Now we're starting from the ground zero of motivation: who I am. This embodies *all* of the important Whys in your life. Your motivation to be a better partner, parent, adult child, professional, caregiver, community member, and/or friend converts your self-care behavior into *essential fuel* for the things that matter most to you. This transforms self-care from simply being a *want* into a *need*, something you feel compelled to fit in and motivated to maintain.

FIGURE 8-2. The Sustainable Cycle of Self-Care.

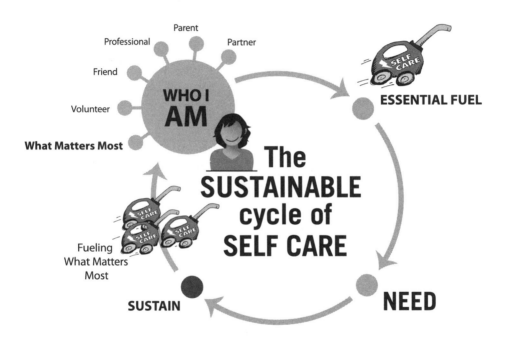

When a self-care behavior becomes a daily need, we *sustain* it. We prioritize it in our lives much more easily, because it helps us with being who we are by *fueling what matters most to us*. Because—and here comes my mantra again—what sustains us, we sustain.[5]

IT'S YOUR MOVE

Assess Your Feelings About Self-Care

Answer the following question by circling the number that best applies:

The idea of doing daily self-care behaviors like getting enough sleep and regular physical activity feels ...

1 2 3 4 5 6 7 8 9 10

Not at all compelling   **Very compelling**

File that away. We'll come back to it.

What Sustains Us, We Sustain

We've been taught to look at our day as a linear progression we go through from waking to sleeping, filled with all of the many things we need to accomplish. But that concept misses something crucial: Our day is actually a dynamic system, a complex interaction of people, goals, meetings, feelings, thoughts, energy, and actions, along with the inevitable unexpected challenges that arise. The key word here is *interaction*: Each of these affects the others. Instead of thinking about how to fit regular physical activity into a crammed schedule, it's much more useful to consider the many ways in which physical activity can help us joyously and resiliently interact with what we care most about.

When psychologists help people create a behavior change, it's common practice to start by asking them about their core values and hoped-for life goals. Yet these are ideals; they are not necessarily urgent needs. They are frequently not relevant to our essential roles and goals and the fires we have to put out on most days. Our daily decisions tend to be based on what is most emotional for us today, not future ideals or aspirations. To help you create the consistent decisions that underlie sustainable behavior, I ask you to work within the very real system of your current daily life: your needs, pains, energy level, and what matters most to you *now*. In order to create consistent, sustainable self-care, it has to be rooted in the realities of our daily life, what we need to do *today*.

Although it often seems that everyday life competes with self-care activities like physical movement, the opposite is true. Consider that regular physical activity *is* revitalizing. It *makes* us feel happier. It *reduces* our stress. It helps us *focus* our minds. It *helps* us resiliently face our challenges and *fuels* our most cherished roles and responsibilities. No, physical activity is not competing with what matters most; it's actually energizing and nurturing it. Figure 8-3 shows a tree that illustrates the daily reality and wisdom of the core message of this book: What sustains us, we sustain.

FIGURE 8-3. The "What Sustains Us, We Sustain" tree.

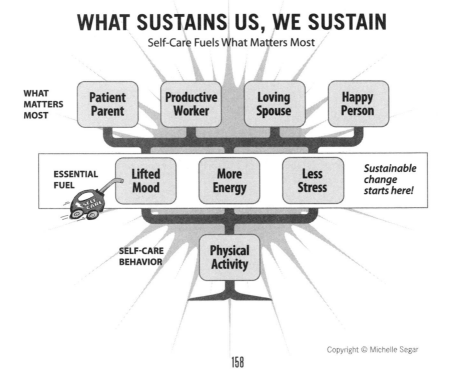

WHAT SUSTAINS US, WE SUSTAIN
Self-Care Fuels What Matters Most

WHAT MATTERS MOST

Patient Parent | Productive Worker | Loving Spouse | Happy Person

ESSENTIAL FUEL

Lifted Mood | More Energy | Less Stress | *Sustainable change starts here!*

SELF-CARE BEHAVIOR

Physical Activity

The base of this tree is grounded in physical activity, the self-care behavior we are focusing on in this book. When you move in ways you like that make you feel good, it generates essential fuel—the positive experiences you need—a lifted mood, more energy, and less stress, as well as other benefits (shown on the middle level) to optimally accomplish the roles and responsibilities that matter most (shown on the highest level of the tree). In other words, physical activity links directly to feeling better and living a meaningful life.

But being physically active in ways that generate positive experiences and meaningful living leads to more than just sustainability. Science also shows that spending time in activities that help us feel good and are personally meaningful also leads to well-being.[6] Consider how this sequential cycle works. When we have well-being and feel good, we are energized to fuel what matters most. When we accomplish our cherished roles and goals, we experience well-being and have more energy. And this self-perpetuating positive cycle just continues to help us expand ourselves and build happier and healthier lives.

Positive Emotions Help Us Build Better Lives

Psychologist Barbara Fredrickson is a pioneer in research seeking to understand the mental and physical health benefits of positive emotions. Her broaden-and-build theory of positive emotions has been gaining support for its proposition that feeling *momentary* positive emotions (from being physically active, spending time with people we enjoy, etc.) broadens us psychologically and physiologically, and this accumulates over time to help us build happier, healthier, and more meaningful lives.[7]

In a review spanning the last fifteen years (as this book goes to press), a growing body of research shows that compared to negative or neutral emotions, positive emotions broaden our thinking and behavior through making us more creative, integrative, flexible, open to information, efficient, and open to others, among other benefits.[8]

Fredrickson's research shows that this psychological broadening helps people regulate negative emotional experiences, have closer relationships, buffer depressive symptoms, and recover better from the stressors of daily life.

Fredrickson's research further shows that under the influence of positive emotions, people's perceptions are more inclusive and their bodies are more relaxed and expansive. She has found that these benefits, in turn, help people build positive trajectories of growth through increased resilience, resourcefulness, and social connectedness and higher levels of optimal functioning. According to her, certain discrete positive emotions—including joy, interest, contentment, pride, and love—although phenomenologically distinct, all share the ability to broaden people's momentary thought-action repertoires and build their enduring personal resources, ranging from physical and intellectual resources to social and psychological resources.[9]

In other words, the daily experiences of positive emotions and meaningful living that we can get from self-care can *broaden us psychologically and even physiologically*—compounding over time to *build* a variety of consequential personal resources, including even better health.[10] Wow. In addition, there is even evidence that experiences that are just pleasurable are also health *promoting*. Research suggests that spending time in hedonic activities that deliver pleasure are health promoting because they are associated with decreased stress and depression.[11] Spending time in pleasant activities is even an evidence-based treatment approach that is prescribed by clinicians to improve health outcomes among patients living with the chronic illness fibromyalgia.[12]

At this point in society, positivity is an underappreciated resource for building well-being, meaning, and health. Thank goodness for research like Fredrickson's and that influential people like Arianna Huffington are creating compelling public conversations about the need to change our norms and expand our definition of a successful life to include living more mindfully, cultivating well-being, and thriving. In fact, Huffington has created an entire section on the Huffington Post website on encouraging others to adopt this paradigm shift, which she calls "The Third Metric."[13]

Are you ready to go from just surviving to thriving? The place to start is by assessing where you are right now.

IT'S YOUR MOVE
Are You Thriving or Just Surviving?

In general, how do you rate your energy level?

1 2 3 4 5 6 7 8 9 10

Low Energy   High Energy

In general, how do you rate your sense of well-being?

1 2 3 4 5 6 7 8 9 10

Low Well-Being   High Well-Being

Are you surprised by your answers? Take a minute, close your eyes, and think about what you are struggling with in your daily life. Go back to Chapter 7 and take a look at the experiences you checked off in your Daily Self-Care Needs Assessment. Consider how physical activity (or some other self-care) might be able to help you realize those experiences. Try it out.

Make sure to repeat this assessment every day or at the same time each week. Ask yourself if your general energy level and well-being are going up. Try to notice whether your scores are higher on the days that you move compared to on the days that you sit most of the day.

What Do I Need Right Now?

For self-care to be a consistent priority, it has to feel more than good. It needs to feel *really compelling* to do. *Right now*.

When Isla (whom you met toward the beginning of this chapter) was starting to figure this out, I suggested she create a list of experiences that would fuel her on a daily basis. This would be, as she later told me:

> A list of as many things I could think of that would feel good to do but also rejuvenate and permit me to recalibrate my energy. I listed things like spending time alone, in nature, with good friends, meditating, listening to music, and painting.
>
> Once I saw how many options I had, I realized two things. First, there was no way I could do all of them every day. But that freed me up to see the second realization: I have a large list of options to choose from every day. I need to pick only one or two, the options that most call to me on that day, and I am able to recalibrate myself. I'm finding it's like ordering from a menu or picking a tool out of a large tool kit. I just have to check in with myself and ask, "What do I need right now?"
>
> I used to have my self-care be contingent on achieving other things, using it like a reward. But it was rare that I made the time that way. I now see that self-care is not my reward—it's actually my daily fuel. It helps me both feel better and be my best. I know this is kind of corny, but it's just like Steven Covey said in his book *First Things First*—you have to put the most important things in first, or other smaller, more urgent things fill up all of the space.

I also asked Isla to come up with a need, an experience that she wanted to enhance on most days—something she was longing to feel. She chose *inspired, energetic, relief, calm,* and *centered.* "That's a lot!" I said. "It's probably best if you pick only one for now to focus on." Isla picked *inspired.* I suggested that she put a reminder on her smartphone to pop up first thing when she got to work to remind her that she wants to live in ways that feel inspiring to her. I also suggested that near the end of the day, she rate from 1 (not at all inspired) to 10 (very inspired) how inspired she felt during that day.

As she recalls, "What I noticed was that by keeping that one need in mind, I was motivated to make decisions that would help me realize it. And then I started seeing how many of these choices actually left me feeling more inspired! After doing this for just a few weeks, my general level of inspiration went up three points (from a 3 to a 6) and it's been a pretty steady 7 to 8. My mindset has changed, I feel better, I am more creative, I do more for others—I am deeply motivated to continue to take good care of myself. Because what I feel like I want or need on any given day changes, I'm also trying to learn how to choose the self-care activity that's right for that day or moment."

The Conundrum:
Which Self-Care Activity Do You Choose?

One day last October, I arranged my schedule so that I could go work at Zingerman's Deli. It's my favorite out-of-office workplace. I get a lot done on my laptop (and eat great food) in a crazy, loud environment that inspires my thinking. On this day, my work was going great and I had some wonderful creative energy going. And then I looked out the window. It was a beautiful fall Michigan day, temperature in the sixties, and the sun was lighting up the red, orange, and yellow leaves on the trees.

Suddenly, I was faced with a choice: Was I going to celebrate this gift of a beautiful day by driving to the Arboretum and taking a walk, or was I going to stay in this cozy place working up until the last minute? Was I going to keep up my intellectually stimulating work in this wonderful place or take up some of my very precious time moving my body?

Yes, I am one of the biggest advocates of physical activity you'll ever meet, but I also love to work. My work deeply nurtures and stimulates me—it's important self-care, too. Frequently, even for me, it's a hard choice to leave work despite knowing that moving my body is such an important self-care activity.

So I was faced with two choices for self-care. Should I keep working and tend to my work/mind self (which I wanted to do in a big way, and I had a lot of work to get done besides)? Or should I pay attention to my physical self (those fall leaves were really calling me)?

What a shame to miss out on the Arb today, I thought. *It's so close, and this is a spectacular day*. At that moment I realized that I had made the choice.

I packed up my laptop and purposefully drove to the Arboretum. Once I let go of to-dos and recommitted to caring for my physical self, the act of moving became kind of sacred. This time wasn't about accomplishing something—it was about honoring being alive and all of the wonderful things in my life.

As I walked through the park, I felt grateful to have access to such a beautiful place for moving. Looking at the river, the trees, and the colors, I felt such deep appreciation. I also felt profoundly moved. After about ten minutes, I turned around, and in another ten I returned to the parking lot. Wow. It was only twenty minutes of walking versus another forty-five minutes of work that I could have ticked off. But when I weighed the real value of these two alternatives on that particular day, there was no contest.

The rest of that day, my walk through the Arb reverberated throughout all my meaningful areas of my life: It generated positive emotions and energy that enabled me to be more appreciative and present with my family, and it even lasted into the next day as optimism toward my upcoming intense work demands. Paradoxically, even though I had not done the work I planned to do (and needed to do that day), I accomplished it after my walk with more ease than I would have thought possible.

Giving ourselves Permission to choose to spend time to feel better over accomplishing more on our to-do list isn't particularly valued in our society, yet it has high pragmatic value. Moving our bodies in an activity we enjoy is exponentially beneficial: It lifts our mood, gives us more energy, enables us to focus better, promotes our immune system, and helps us to sleep better, all of which join together and enable us to enjoy our work more and be more loving to our loved ones.

Here's the deal: We hit decision points about choosing to take better care of ourselves, through moving or other activities, almost every day. Choosing to move isn't always going to be the right choice. As I write these words now, I'm choosing to finish this book instead of walking outside on another particularly beautiful Michigan day. What we choose every day depends upon what's going on, who needs what, and deadlines that need to be met. The challenge we all face in that moment is to determine what's most important for us to do *in that moment*.

Sometimes we make the best choice, and sometimes we don't. Check in with yourself at the point of decision. Ask yourself a frank question: What do I *most* need right now? Is it to get more done, or is it to give to myself in some way? Then, sometime later that day or night, notice if you feel any regret about your decision or whether, deep down, you *know* that, for that day, your choice was the right one.

I have choices that I later regret on many occasions. At these times, I remind myself that it's a learning curve. Then I try to recall those "wrong" decision moments every time I find myself at the point of decision, and I do my best to make the right choice that day.

Self-care isn't optional, something we do if we have an extra hour in our day. Getting enough sleep, moving in enjoyable ways every day—these and other self-care behaviors are essential to our daily functioning and to fostering what matters most. Our daily decisions and behaviors embody our priorities; they grow out of what we value and what we believe is important. We can sustain daily self-care and physical activity much better *if* we've chosen it because it helps us to feel good and reflects who we genuinely are and what matters most.

IT'S YOUR MOVE

Checking In on Your Priorities by Revisiting Your Personal Projects List

Now that we've discussed how essential self-care is to fuel what matters most in your life, it's time to become aware of where self-care has sat in your life among your life projects and priorities and assess if you want it to stay there or not. Go back and revisit the list of personal projects you made at the end of Chapter 1. Take a moment to review your responses, and then think about these questions:

1. Among your top five personal projects, did you list any project related to "having a sense of well-being" or "taking good care of myself"? *Yes / No*

2. If you answered No to question 1, would you like to try giving yourself Permission to make creating your own quality of life and/or self-care one of your top personal projects so it is among your top daily priorities? If you would, why? If you don't want to right now, why not?

3. If you answered Yes to question 1, based on what you've read in this book so far, what do you feel is a good next step to advancing your own self-care and well-being?

4. Review your answer to the question posed earlier in this chapter about how compelling you found the idea of doing daily self-care behaviors like getting enough sleep and regular physical activity. Would you change your answer in any way now? If so, in what direction?

This final chapter in the Permission part of the book is the integration and culmination of all of the chapters about Meaning, Awareness, and Permission—your MAP. Now it's time to take your personal MAP and move on to the final part of this book: Strategy. In fact, you already know one *big* Strategy: Being physically active is itself a *specific Strategy* to fuel your daily functioning and performance. Now it's time to take that ball and run (or walk at an enjoyable pace) with it. The chapters in the Strategy part will guide you through the logistics of self-regulation and goal pursuit, providing specific negotiation Strategies, skills, and tools you can use to integrate physical activity into your life and create a sustainable source of energy and joy for what matters most.

The Takeaways

- The self-care paradox reflects the idea that the more energy you give to caring for yourself, the more energy you have to give to and fuel what matters most in your life.

- Self-care helps you with being fully yourself, a parent, a partner, and a professional, and brings you well-being.

- Permission to prioritize self-care transforms it from a gift into your essential fuel.

- When you spend time in activities that are meaningful and generate positive emotions and experiences, (e.g., physical activities you enjoy), it increases meaning, resilience, and well-being.

- In order to integrate physical movement and self-care into the rest of your life, it needs to feel compelling and play a meaningful role in your daily life. Try to consider your own self-care and well-being one of your top personal projects.

- Regular physical activity is revitalizing, makes you feel happier and more resilient, and fuels your most cherished roles and responsibilities.

- The Sustainable Cycle of Self-Care begins when you choose a self-care behavior to help you with being who you are and to fuel what matters most in your life. What sustains us, we sustain.

- Research on the broaden-and-build theory of positive emotions shows that experiences of momentary positive emotions broaden people psychologically and physiologically, accumulating over time to help them build happier, healthier, and more resilient and meaningful lives.

PART IV

• • • • •

STRATEGY

Use learning and negotiation STRATEGIES to
sustain the lifelong gift of physical activity.

9

Six Big Ideas for Lifelong Sustainability

AT THE BEGINNING OF OUR SECOND SESSION, EMILY, A FINANCIAL adviser in her thirties, was overflowing with excitement. "Michelle, I exercised for fifty minutes every day for six days last week! I'm so happy with myself!"

Uh-oh.

"I don't want to burst your bubble," I said, "but that's a red flag for me."

"What are you talking about? It was great!"

"It's great that you had such a good time," I said, "but we're playing a long game here—a *lifetime*. And that kind of sustainable success won't be based on you exercising six days a week for fifty minutes, or seven days a week for half an hour, or whatever arbitrary goals you want to achieve. It will be a result of how much you like what you're doing, how you're interacting with challenges to your plans, and how creative you can be about finding opportunities to move even when your schedule seems most crammed. Is this making sense?"

Silence.

I pressed on. "It's not *how much* you exercise in any given week—it's whether you have the mindset and Strategies to interact with and improvise with the ebbs and flows of things so you are still consistently moving years from now."

"But this was the best week of working out I've ever had!" Emily protested. "You mean I *shouldn't* keep working out six days a week?"

"If you're having fun, that's great. But realistically, you probably can't count on getting in six free fifty-minute time segments every week forever without life somehow getting in the way. And then what? What happens when you miss a workout? How are you going to bounce back and get back on track?"

Emily was quiet, taking it all in.

"Perfection isn't the goal. Just take every challenge as it comes, see how many ways you can negotiate with it, and discover how many different ways you can find to give your body a chance to move. Some will be fun; others can just be a pragmatic opportunity to keep moving. Look, your objective is to keep this up for life, right?"

"Right . . ."

"Well, life is a moving target. It doesn't stop so that you can work out when you planned," I said. "Don't get ahead of yourself, trying to do it all, and then be disappointed when things don't work out. Aiming to achieve a perfect outcome every week sets people up for disappointment and even stopping altogether. Instead, try having a learning mindset. Respect that you are in a process of learning something new, and enjoy the trial and error—you're learning skills that will allow you to reap a lifetime of benefits. Experiment with new Strategies and attitudes to overcome the challenges that arise to your plans. Let yourself learn how to become consistent by starting small. Then, as you begin to feel confident that you can overcome these barriers, start increasing what you want to do by modest amounts. Sometimes you'll do five or six intense workouts a week, sometimes you won't. But as long as you keep moving, you're on the right track."

My conversation with Emily embodies one of the most important messages in this book: When your objective is to maintain consistent physical movement for a lifetime, you need to appreciate that you are in an actual learning process and become comfortable using Strategies that will help you find ways to be resilient and successful in the face of the many challenges that never stop arising to your ongoing pursuit of a lifetime of being happy, healthy, and fit.

With a learning mindset, setbacks and failures don't enter the picture. They are naturally reframed as opportunities we mindfully learn from. The first time a child touches a hot stove, she doesn't consider herself a failure—she simply learns not to touch the hot stove again. She adds that bit of learning to her lifetime store of knowledge and then moves right on to something else. In this mindset, we're not sapping energy by adding up our failures but fueling ourselves with the positive energy that comes from figuring out new ways we can do things. We discover Strategies and build skills and resilience that we can use when we inevitably encounter new challenges in the future. And it can even be fun because we get to be creative when we devise novel ways to negotiate with our challenges.

In real life, the behaviors necessary to achieve and sustain the outcomes we want are very complex. Changing our eating habits or integrating exercise into a busy life are not simple tasks, as you undoubtedly already know. It's tempting to look to any specific outcome we want to achieve, like improving our cholesterol by a certain number of points, as success—proof that our efforts have worked. But focusing on achieving specific outcomes won't help us sustain our success. Instead, long-term success necessitates focusing on learning how to sustain the behaviors that *create* our desired outcomes.

Learning redirects us from achieving arbitrary goals to engaging with "learning goals," mastering new tasks such as learning how to be active for fifteen minutes on most days is a good first step. This perspective asks us to discover the steps we need to take to integrate and sustain a new behavior in our busy lives, and to consider the other options we did not know we had. By guiding you to discover the Strategies, processes, and procedures necessary to do any task or behavior effectively, learning goals will help you master the task rather than stress over achieving a specific goal. The six Big Ideas in this chapter provide a high-level framework for the ten negotiation Strategies presented in Chapter 10. Together, they will help you integrate physical activity and self-care into your life consistently and confidently, so that you successfully negotiate the challenges that each day brings.

Big Idea #1: Use Learning Goals to Get Intrinsic Motivation, Persistence, and Resilience

This is not just a good idea to consider but a fundamental one. An extraordinary amount of research in the field of education has looked at which is more motivationally potent: a *performance* goal, like exercising five times a week, or a *learning* goal, like discovering how to stay consistently physically active. Data from leading motivation psychologist Carol Dweck's laboratory strongly shows that a learning mindset—approaching life with a genuine curiosity about making discoveries and learning new ways of doing things—results in more internal motivation and greater persistence and resilience in the face of challenges.[1]

This makes sense. When our goal is to learn, we are naturally curious and interested and want to pay attention when challenges arise. It's easy to see why being curious actually raises our Awareness and motivates us to discover more creative and flexible Strategies in the face of challenges.

Many of these powerful ideas from Dweck's laboratory are supported by findings from researchers in a much different area: performance at work. For example, Edwin Locke and Gary Latham have spent the last three decades studying which types of goals lead to better or worse performance under different conditions.[2] Like Dweck, they have similarly investigated the influence of learning goals on performance and outcomes. Interestingly, their research also shows that when a task is complex (like physical activity) and environments are dynamic (like daily life), having a learning perspective is key for an optimal outcome.[3] They note that when people focus on achieving a *specific* goal (lower cholesterol, losing weight) with a new, complex behavior (sustaining a physically active life), it leads to "tunnel vision"—an overfocus on reaching the goal instead of acquiring the *skills* required to reach it and sustain it.

These independent programs of research over decades strongly support the wisdom of having your goal be to *learn* how you can sustain life-enhancing daily movement within your busy, ever-changing life. Shifting to a learning mindset is an important concept that underlies all of the more specific Strategies you will learn.

Big Idea #2: Begin with the End in Mind

Let's get this out of the way right now: Health and fitness solutions touting quick fixes are false promises that sound exciting and get our hopes up but quickly lead us down a road that detours into disappointment and a sense of failure. Anyone who tells you there really *is* a magic bullet when it comes to lifelong behavior change is, frankly, full of crap.

Consider that your learning goal is the *ongoing pursuit* of a lifetime of consistent physical movement and self-care. It's more than just a turn of phrase: It reflects your desire and ability to maintain movement as a part of your hectic life. Life is never stagnant, and as you know by now, we can't really predict or control it. If you are going to be successful staying physically active and taking care of yourself, you need to learn Strategies that will enable you to prioritize your plans and be consistent, flexible, and creative as you learn to incorporate physical activity into the rest of your dynamic, ever-changing life.

The Strategy of beginning with the end in mind asks you to take the long view: Your goal is lifelong behavior change, and that's what you want to keep in mind—always. This really puts the issue in perspective! When we want to stick with something for life, we start asking different questions and looking for more in return. I often think of this shift in perspective as similar to moving from the highs and lows of casual dating to discovering the person you want to spend the rest of your life with.

I remember what happened when I suggested this dating analogy to Beth, a client in her mid-fifties who was married for the second time, this time to a much more suitable partner. She burst out laughing after I said it. "Beth," I went on, "consider the parallels. When you're dating, your attention is focused on excitement, the rush, someone you can have a lot of fun with. But when you're ready to find a partner for life, the criteria drastically change. You still want to have fun and feel sexy, but there are bigger questions that relate to a lifetime: Will this person be there for me when I'm going through a rough time? Will this person be a loving, patient parent if we decide to have children?"

Beth nodded in agreement. "I see what you're getting at."

"The marketing from fitness companies has educated us to approach exercise as if we were dating it," I went on, "seeking the rush of the next new thing that will help us lose weight or look fabulous or please our doctors. But in reality, we need the steady partner who will stick with us, have fun with us, and give us the support we need throughout life."

She laughed again. "Maybe if I'd spoken to you about this idea when I was in my twenties, I would have taken better care of myself for the last thirty years—and I wouldn't have married that jerk Frank, either!"

Here's the difference between taking a short-term and long-term view of being physically active: When you have a short-term goal to, say, achieve a weight loss of ten pounds, you find yourself calculating how many calories you're burning in twenty minutes on the treadmill or forty minutes of boot camp. When you lose the weight, you're done. What will keep you motivated once you reach your goal if that was your focus? Or if your progress slows toward that goal, will you stay motivated to keep it up? But when your goal is a lifetime of physical movement, you take the long view. Now, every step you take is a genuine step toward self-care and well-being. Even though you might make weekly plans, your horizon is the rest of your life. Whether you are walking, running, playing tennis, riding a bike, dancing, or climbing the stairs to make the bed, you are progressing on your path. Knowing that is true helps you feel successful and reinforces your greater goal.

Big Idea #3: Use Sustainable Self-Care as an Essential Strategy for Well-Being

You've probably heard tactics such as "put your oxygen mask on first" or "you need to manage your energy." While good advice, these ideas don't really get to the heart of the matter because they don't explicitly address the really compelling reason, or Why. In contrast, this Big Idea cuts to the quick and directly showcases the huge return on investment when you consistently prioritize your own self-care. When we purposively use a self-care behavior like physical movement to help us feel and be better, it simultaneously turns that behavior into both a powerful reward and a personally meaningful act that helps us with *being* who we are more fully. As previously mentioned, there are different but synergistic effects from spending time in activities that deliver positive experiences and also feel meaningful; these two distinct experiences build upon and amplify each other in sequential ways, thus expanding our experience of well-being. Feeling positive and energetic gives us more energy for the roles and responsibilities we care most about. When we work toward what is most meaningful, we generate positive emotions, continually expanding our sense of well-being and nurturing our sense of self.

So now you know the secret: Using physical activity as a Strategy to generate both positive experiences and meaningful living does much more than just put us into the Sustainable Cycle of Self-Care. It also creates an amplifying growth cycle that guides us right onto what I call the Expanding Path of Well-Being (Figure 9-1).

FIGURE 9-1. The Expanding Path of Well-Being.

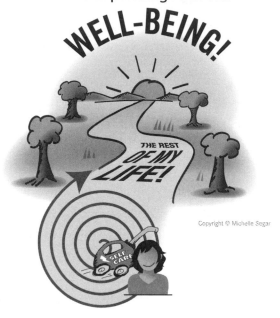

As you can see, sustaining self-care is among the most strategic things you can do to feel happy as you strive toward the personal projects that you care most about every day.

Big Idea #4: Integrate One New Behavior at a Time

Two years after our first conversation, my client Nolan told me, "You know, Michelle, I was very skeptical of your suggestion that I focus on learning only one new behavior at a time, but that turned out to be such an important Strategy for me." Like many of my clients, Nolan came to me impatient and geared up to make *mountainous* change in behavior. He was ready to completely overhaul his eating habits and exercise routines at the same time—again. It wouldn't be the first time he'd tried and failed. So when I suggested he might give another Strategy a try, he was open to it.

As you learned in our discussion of willpower in Chapter 2, we have a finite store of mental energy. And because we all juggle multiple roles and responsibilities, we have a limited amount of additional time and attention besides. Our mental energy gets depleted with every decision we make—more so if we need to make a difficult choice or exert self-control in a really tough situation or if we give ourselves multiple new tasks to learn at the same time. Given our limited cognitive resources, the smartest thing we can do is let ourselves focus on learning how to integrate and sustain only one new behavior at a time.*

Your long-term goal is to learn how to integrate consistent movement into each day for the rest of your life, but you can't do it all in a day or a week or a month. Take your time and enjoy the journey. Take a month or two now to learn how to add five or ten minutes of physical activity to your life on most days. Then, once you've mastered learning that specific thing, ramp up the time or change what you are doing and give yourself another three to six months to feel comfortable and confident doing that. You've got your whole life to be active. Why not take sufficient time to learn how to sustain it?

Big Idea #5: Strengthen the Core— Build Consistency Before Quantity

A big reason that people find it difficult to sustain a physically active life is because they are too ambitious and try to do too much in the beginning. Like brushing your teeth every day, the real key to sustain-

---

* That said, there is an exception to every rule: You may have a specific medical situation that mandates changing more than one behavior at once. If you have a health concern, you should work with your healthcare provider to identify how to optimally manage it. In addition, physical activity is known to be helpful when quitting smoking, so becoming physically active while you quit might be a good Strategy to try, even though it involves two different changes at once.

ing self-care and a physically active life is being consistent. Consistency is the core stabilizer of sustainability. So let's focus on strengthening the core!

When I was a kid, we learned how to ride bikes by using training wheels as the first step. A few years later, someone figured out that it's not pedaling that's the hard part to learn about biking—it's balancing on the bike. Last year, when we taught our son to ride his bike, he started off with a balance bike—a bike without pedals. He learned to balance his body and get comfortable in this easier, pre-pedaling situation. Once he felt comfortable balancing his body on the bike, lifting his legs up as he gained confidence and comfort, we transitioned him to a bike with pedals. Because he already had his core balance, the transition was pretty effortless.

If you are going to learn how to balance physical activity within your life, the most strategic thing you can do is create small, realistic plans that you can more easily learn how to navigate. For example, mindfully choosing to add even an additional five minutes of physical activity into every day, if that's all you feel you have time for, will slowly build the realization that you *can* fit it in. And when you understand how to do that small amount consistently, you can think about ways to fit in a little bit more.

Creating lifelong behavior is your goal, so your focus needs to be on learning how physical activity can fit and *stay* in your busy life. And that's not an easy task. People who join a gym and start out with modest plans to attend just a couple of days a week are more likely to keep coming and stay members than those who begin with grandiose plans to come every day during the first couple of weeks. If you are seeking a *lifetime* of fitness, it's important to start smart.

The speed and complexity of our lives makes adding some large, new thing very difficult. Sure, we can shove it into our lives for a while, but keeping it there takes a great deal of energy and attention. We have great intentions. We always start out strong. But beginning to maintain a new and challenging behavior like exercise, a different diet, or better time management in our crazy, busy lives feels like trying to keep a cow from flying out of a spinning tornado. Eventually, we just watch it fly.

The same challenges are going to arise no matter how large or small your plan. Learning how to overcome challenges with smaller, weekly behavioral goals follows accepted learning principles—that is, it works!—and makes the path to lasting change a more positive and easier experience.

Big Idea #6: Bring Your Learning to Life

To really change your behavior in sustainable ways means moving from theory to practice: taking the concepts you've learned in reading this book, and what you've learned about your beliefs and yourself more generally from the *It's Your Move* exercises you've done so far, and bringing it all to life in the complexity and challenges of day-to-day living.

This idea is based on the work of the renowned Brazilian educator and philosopher Paulo Freire. When I began studying how to help people achieve lifelong behavior change, I was inspired and influenced by his work. Freire believed that "through learning [women and men] can make and remake themselves, because [they] are able to take responsibility for themselves as beings capable of knowing—of knowing that they know and knowing that they don't."[4]

Freire's empowerment-based education method assumes that we need to learn through doing within the reality of our own life. Only then can we truly understand the multiple levels of challenges we have to whatever behavior we want to change—in this case, adopting a physically active life. According to Freire's way of thinking, it is crucial that you view your physical activity and self-care as occurring *within the many contexts of your life*, your mindset, your body, your family, your work, your home, your community, and even the greater society. He also suggests that people who are learning should consider themselves as "beings in the process of becoming—as unfinished, uncompleted beings in a reality that is likewise unfinished and becoming."[5] In the same way, I ask you to consider learning how to integrate physical activity within your daily life as a process that will help you develop the beliefs, insights, self-awareness, drive, personal responsibility, and negotiation skills necessary for you to sustain a physically active life and enjoy living to the fullest.

Instead of wanting to be active "in theory" or being a passive recipient of knowledge (just learning the physical activity recommendations), this approach will lead you to new insights about physical activity *for you* as you work with being physically active in your actual life contexts. Freire calls this learning through action, or *praxis*. Now you are not just being physically active—you are being physically active within the realities of your life, critically reflecting upon your beliefs and expectations, what you learn from doing, and using that learning to further expand what you know. When you approach learning in this way, this expansive process actually helps you become more fully who you are. It's incredibly empowering and exciting.

Now that you have given yourself Permission to prioritize your own self-care as essential fuel, and you've learned the six Big Ideas to orient you to Strategy, you are ready for your sustainability training—the specific Strategies you'll use to negotiate your physical movement, self-care, and well-being throughout the rest of your very busy life.

The Takeaways

• There are six Big Ideas that will create the context for successfully negotiating physical activity within your busy life and cultivating lifelong sustainability.

• When your objective is to maintain consistent physical movement for a lifetime, you need to appreciate that you are in an actual learning process and become comfortable using Strategies that will help you find ways to be resilient and successful in the face of challenges.

- Having a learning mindset and goals will lead you to intrinsic motivation, persistence, and resilience so you can better sustain your behavioral and well-being aims.

- The Strategy of beginning with the end in mind asks you to take the long view. When you want to stick with something for life, you start asking different questions and looking for more in return.

- Use sustainable self-care as an essential Strategy for well-being. Feeling positive and energetic gives you more energy for what you care most about. When you work toward what is most meaningful, you are guided right onto the Expanding Path of Well-Being.

- Given your limited cognitive resources, it is strategic to focus on learning how to integrate and sustain only one new, complex behavior at a time, unless there are medical reasons for doing multiple behavioral changes.

- You should build consistency before quantity to strengthen the core stabilizer of sustainability. If creating lifelong behavior is your goal, your focus should be on learning how physical activity can fit and *stay* in your busy life.

- Bring your learning to life. Learning how to integrate physical activity within your daily life is a process that will help you develop the beliefs, insights, self-awareness, drive, personal responsibility, and negotiation skills necessary for you to sustain a physically active life and enjoy living to the fullest.

10

Sustainability Training

"I CAN'T GET THE HANG OF THIS," SAID JULES. SHE SOUNDED SO MOURN-ful. "I have an app for my physical activity, I put it on the calendar, I have every intention of doing it, and something always gets in my way. Like on Saturday evening, when I was almost out the door to go for a jog, my daughter suddenly decides she needs to come home early from her sleepover, so of course I needed to go pick her up instead. And then on Tuesday morning, when I was all set to get up early and take a walk before breakfast? It was pouring! I almost postponed our session today because honestly, I have so many things to do I couldn't see how I could do this too. I never noticed before how many *obstacles* there are to just taking care of myself!"

Jules had just come up against the hard edge of her transition from theory to practice: She understood that physical activity really does provide fuel for what matters most, and she'd given herself

Permission to make it a priority. She just couldn't figure out how to make that ideal real. "That's not so surprising," I said. "If you think about it, you've never learned how to do this before. Effectively negotiating the never-ending onslaught of challenges is kind of like juggling: It takes getting used to as well as some new skills. Remember when we talked about learning by doing? Well, this is where the rubber hits the road."

No matter how carefully we plan our week, dutifully scheduling in time for exercise, we inevitably encounter an unexpected call for our attention—a sudden change in a friend's plans, an urgent last-minute request from our boss, a sick child who needs to stay home from school, a meeting we *must* attend, a pop quiz to study for. We may spend a week or two happily checking off the days we went to the gym, but Figure 10-1 illustrates how quickly the self-care priorities on our carefully constructed daily schedules get crowded out by other important daily to-dos.

In each moment, we must make choices about which calls to heed and which to disregard. We vow that we're going to stay physically active because it makes us feel good and gives us energy for all the things we need to get done during the day. But even when we deeply want to be physically active, the currents of real life are so strong that they easily overpower even the most autonomous of intentions. As you try to adopt a new behavior like physical activity, it is important to understand that you are trying to do this within the context of your many other valuable daily roles and choices:

» Should I take my child to school (good parent) or go for an early-morning swim (self-care)?

» Should I get to work and finish that report (effective worker) or walk for half an hour (self-care)?

» Should I call Mom (good child) or make dinner for the family (good parent, good partner, good provider) or go to dance class (self-care)?

FIGURE 10-1. How self-care gets crowded out of the day.

OUR PLANS

REALITY

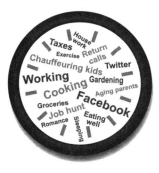

And how we *feel* about our different priorities and goals—regardless of their objective "rightness" or "wrongness"—seems to determine which ones we choose.

Now you have a new long-term goal: to make physical activity and self-care a sustainable and empowering part of your life. But believe it or not, even having this meaningful, autonomous goal isn't necessarily enough to make it happen. We embrace our new self-care goals with enthusiasm when we first commit to them, but competing demands and real-time to-dos are a constant reality that even our cherished goals are always vulnerable to.

Knowing where we want to go is one thing; pursuing that goal and sticking to it, in the context of our very busy lives, is quite another. The first important point to remember is that *we* have goals—goals don't have us. The next stop in this journey is to learn how to effectively negotiate your goals within the complexities of your life each and every day.

Negotiating the Reality of Our Complex and Busy Lives

We are accustomed to thinking of negotiating as something that business executives and attorneys do or something we do when we ask for a raise. But as Shirli Kopelman says in *Negotiating Genuinely*, we negotiate all day long in the different contexts of our lives[1]: with our kids about their bedtime, with our parents about when we can accompany them to the store, with our friends about which restaurant to go to. And we negotiate with ourselves all the time about which of our daily activities, which calls on our time by friends and family and work, and which of our own needs is going to get priority this moment. It's rarely an easy task, but it is a skill you can get better at. In this chapter, I'm going to teach you the negotiation tactics that I teach my clients. In health and wellness contexts, the set of processes you'll learn in this chapter are referred to as *self-regulation*.

The Lynchpin of Sustainability: Self-Regulation and Negotiation

Self-regulation is the way we manage ourselves and our behavior to support our definition of who we are or would like to be. Social psychologists Esther K. Papies and Henk Aarts note that self-regulation is *"the exertion of control over the self by the self,* which involves altering the way an individual feels, thinks or behaves in order to pursue short- or long-term interests [emphasis added]."[2] Self-regulation puts us in control of what we want to do and how we want to do it, the daily processes that we use to steer our thoughts, emotions, and behavior so we achieve our desired goals. Because of that, self-regulation is truly the lynchpin of sustainability.

You already know that research supports autonomous motivation as the key for long-term behavior. But what's really interesting is *how* having autonomous reasons or goals for exercising actually leads to better behavioral pursuit and more exercise. My colleagues and I conducted a study to examine this question,[3] and the year our study was published, I serendipitously discovered that another research group had independently investigated the same general question using distinct methods and studying a very different population.[4] Despite these differences, we generally found the same thing: that people whose goals for exercising were more autonomous (e.g., to feel better) compared to controlled (e.g., to lose weight) exercised more *because they better planned and prioritized it among their other daily goals though self-regulation techniques.*

Wow! This research suggests that when we choose to move with the goal of fueling our daily functioning and performance, it makes it meaningful. Because of that, we are more *committed* to physical activity and motivated to plan it into our schedule and *negotiate* the challenges that arise. In fact, our behavioral goals, or our reasons for being physically active, are considered to be the *hub* of the self-regulatory processes we use in adopting and sustaining new behaviors. When our behavior aims to achieve something meaningful, we want to protect it from challenges, which translates into doing it. Put another way: *Self-regulation is our meaningful motivation manifested.*

The best self-regulation embodies autonomy, desire, energy, and fuel. Meaning, Awareness, and Permission gave you a MAP to a new destination and the resources to fuel and motivate yourself. The only thing missing are the Strategies and skills to navigate and improvise physical activity in your life so you can stick with it through the challenging times. To stay on this new path and keep striving toward your new destination, you need to become more cognizant of what really gets in your way and learn the attitudes and Strategies that will keep you flexible enough to effectively self-regulate, to negotiate physical activity within your ever-changing life.

Sustainability Training for Life

Pilots get training to become skilled in overcoming the issues that likely present challenges to a successful flight, so why shouldn't we? I consider the Strategies outlined in this chapter as *sustainability training, to maintain meaningful physical movement for life.*

My conversation with Jules hinted at the sustainability training that I was going to give her. I'm going to discuss this training in the rest of this chapter. It will help you become comfortable and confident with the mindset and skill set you'll use to successfully make your plans, reconcile all of your valued goals, navigate your hectic schedule, and build support to ensure that your own physical activity and self-care stay embedded in your days and remain a top priority for the rest of your life. Having effective negotiation Strategies puts you in control. You are empowered to try new Strategies, flex a goal one way and then another, see what you like, and see what works and doesn't work. Then, with this heightened Awareness, you can determine the best, most effective Strategies you can use to make your long-term goal your ally and a reality.

This time, you won't be starting yet another new self-care behavior on faith that you will finally get it right, and you won't be trying to cram it into the nooks and crannies of your life when New Year's Eve brings you a burst of motivation. Rather, when you decide to learn negotiation Strategies, you take the reins—setting up the systems that help you make the consistent decisions that enable you to flourish while you mindfully manage your many daily roles and goals.

Become a Skilled Self-Care Negotiator

Understanding what you want to get out of physical activity, planning what you're going to do, previewing your potential challenges, monitoring what happens, mindfully negotiating with your challenges, and evaluating how it all went constitutes my sustainability training, what I am going to refer to as "negotiation" throughout this chapter. It reflects an Awareness-raising comprehensive system of evidence-based and practical Strategies you can use to figure out what's working for you and what isn't, so that you can use different Strategies as needed. Regular planning and monitoring like this really helps people learn the self-regulation processes for sustaining a new behavior.

No one is born with all of the resilience and coping skills needed to negotiate life, but you can always learn them. Give yourself Permission to actively participate in setting your own pace; choosing your expectations, experiences, and plans; reframing obstacles as challenges and then approaching them with curiosity, flexibility, and creativity; and evaluating and then tweaking your program to make it fit your life. Negotiating lets you work *with* instead of *against* the realities of your life.

My client Chris still plans her weekly negotiations long after we stopped working together. She explains, "Now, at the beginning of each week, I decide what I want from it and for the most part I now get it. Michelle, when you originally explained to me that this is similar to a business having a vision or mission, a lightbulb went on in my brain. By shining a bright light on the specifics of what I want each week ahead of time, I am more likely to align my daily decisions so that they realize those very objectives. It made perfect sense when you explained this to me, and I've found it really works in practice."

Make a Self-Care Negotiation Plan

My version of self-care negotiation is the whole shebang: all of the parts working together as a system. To explain how it works, the rest of this chapter is divided into the three primary phases that reflect the way I train my clients in effective self-care negotiation: (1) Planning and Previewing, (2) Negotiation in Action, and (3) Nonjudgmental Evaluation and Recalibration.

Phase 1: Planning and Previewing

You'll be more likely to get your needs met if you preview what you want to get out of being physically active, plan it into your schedule, and anticipate the likely scenarios you'll need to negotiate. If you feel like you don't have any time to begin with, taking time to create a plan may seem like more trouble than it's worth. In fact, the opposite is true. When you are just beginning to adopt a physically active life (or any other self-care behavior), it pays *big time* to think about your upcoming week and create a plan of action. It's not until we actually sit down with concrete plans that we can see what challenges arise. Once we understand the types of things that tend to get in the way of our plans, we can start using our negotiation Strategies on them.

Even if you're thinking "I've made plans before, and they never work," please give this system a try.

Negotiation Strategy #1: Give Physical Activity Clout

The first negotiation Strategy is about understanding the specific value that movement brings to our daily lives, giving it influence—or clout— within the dynamics of all of your other daily roles and goals. I coined the term *giving physical activity clout* as a deceptively simple and extremely effective Strategy that I use all the time. Basically, we're doubling up, even tripling up, on behaviors, consciously using physical activity to aid in accomplishing other things that we care about—in one small swoop. For example, when I park twenty minutes away from work in order to get in a walk that day, it facilitates spending time outside, fitting in movement, and saving money (since there's no need to pay for parking like I have to if I park near my office).

I enjoy recognizing the multiple benefits I get from the same twenty minutes and give myself points for the strategic nature of this walk. But these concurrent perks are not the core reason for my movement. Instead, it's my belief (gained from my experience) that regular physical movement is a very effective way to ignite the energy, confidence, and enthusiasm that helps me be myself fully as I joyfully work on my most meaningful personal projects. When we recognize the concrete ways that physical activity revitalizes us so we can fuel what matters most every day, it has clout! Remember the "What Sustains Us, We Sustain" tree in Figure 8-3? This is what I'm talking about.

If our physical activity isn't filled with value from the beginning, it won't make the cut when all our other life tasks start crowding in. Dr. Winnie Gebhardt and her colleagues advocate making physical activity (or any behavior) more relevant and compelling to your daily life by linking it to what matters most in your life, a Strategy officially called *goal facilitation*.[5] The "What Sustains Us, We Sustain" tree shown in Figure 10-2 is a blank template that you can fill in based on your daily wants and needs.

People commonly think that the best place to start a behavior change process is at the top, by defining what matters most, or at the bottom, by identifying and scheduling self-care behaviors. But I've found that *neither* is the best place to start to turn self-care into an integral and sustainable part of our daily life. The best place to focus on first is in the *middle* of the tree, where our energy—our essential fuel—resides. Understanding the very real links between these positive emotional experiences in the middle level is what "hooks" us, getting us to *like* and keep *wanting* it again and again (just like the neuroscience of reward discussed in Chapter 6). After we successfully establish this core motivational link with being active, we can then turn our attention to understanding the subsequent link to what matters most.

In Chapter 8, Isla had many different experiences she wanted to have in her day, but I asked her to focus on only one in the beginning. Similarly, after you fill out the tree, you should circle the *single* posi-

FIGURE 10-2. Blank "What Sustains Us, We Sustain" tree.

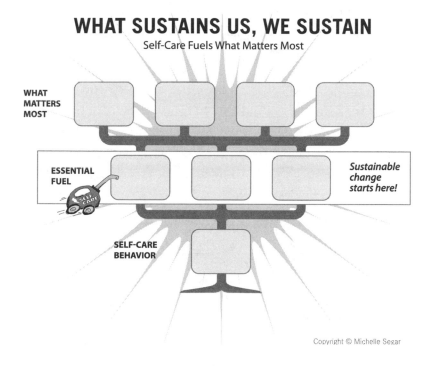

tive experience (e.g., type of essential fuel) you are most in need of having from being active this week. Especially when we are just starting out, it is helpful to focus our attention on creating an association between physical activity and one experience that will most help us fulfill our daily self-care needs. Giving physical activity clout necessitates that you first lay out the specific ways movement infuses your daily life with energy and meaning. Experiencing the strong influence physical activity has gives it the clout needed to trump the unexpected challenges that may potentially get in its way.

Negotiation Strategy #2: Plan the Weekly Logistics

Once you've given your physical activity clout, imbuing it with positivity and purpose for your daily life, you can move on to planning the logistical issues. This part of the planning process deals with pragmatic questions: What physical activities will help me realize the benefits I want? When will I do them? For how long? Where?

Use the worksheet below to address all of the logistical planning. Here are the steps:

1. Determine which physical activities will help you realize the essential experiences and benefits you desire. (Choose to move in ways that will deliver what you want to experience and gain.) Figure out when you can fit these activities into your week. (And remember to give yourself explicit Permission to prioritize your own self-care.)

2. When will you do these activities, where, with whom, and for how long?

3. Create your continuum of success.

You're likely wondering what I mean by "continuum of success." Research shows that people are more successful at achieving their goals when they can choose from a range of low-end and high-end goals rather than aiming at one specific goal.[6] For example, your low end might be "Fit in *one* of my planned activities," and your high end might be "Fit in *all* of my planned activities." *Anywhere you land on that continuum is a success.*

I love this idea because when we feel successful being physically active, it positively influences our performance perceptions, including how we feel during and afterward.[7] A positive perception boosts our confidence, motivation, and participation; why fail if you don't have to? Creating a personalized range of activities that permits success at many points can help increase your confidence and help you develop positive feelings about your abilities and being physically active. If you do one minute, you can do two . . . and who knows what else you can do? But I guarantee it will be fun to find out.

Use this worksheet at the beginning of every week to plan your physical activities.

WEEKLY PHYSICAL ACTIVITY
NEGOTIATION PLANNING WORKSHEET

KEY QUESTIONS	EXAMPLES
This week, I'd like to have the following experience/feeling in order to fuel my week and enhance my sense of well-being:	*I'd like to feel energized.*
What areas of my daily life do I want to fuel through being physically active?	*I want to be fueled to be more patient with my son, more present with my husband, and more focused at work.*
What physical activities can I plan this week that will deliver those experiences?	*yoga, walking*
What Permissions do I need to give myself in order to make this plan happen?	*I give myself Permission to get takeout for dinner instead of cooking so that I can get to yoga class.*
When will I do it?	*Take a class on Wednesday night; do a video at home before work on Friday; walk on Saturday and Sunday*
Where will I do it?	*The Y; practice in the living room; walk in my neighborhood*
How long do I want to do it for?	*1 hour for class, plus 15 minutes to get there and back; 10 minutes in the morning; 45 minutes each weekend day*
What is my continuum of success this week (my low, high, and middle range of activities)?	*My low end is doing just one of the three planned physical activities above. My high end is doing all of the activities above. My middle range is doing at least one of the planned activities plus searching out and choosing every OTM I can find, such as taking the Long Cut to places.*

Negotiation Strategy #3: Decide to Confront Challenges, Not Roadblocks

Roadblocks get in our way and prevent us from achieving our plans. They present us with either-or choices: Either we get around this roadblock, or we don't get to do our activity. This is a very limited point of view, and it is no help at all in dealing with the many curve-balls that are thrown at our schedules every day. So I propose doing something completely different. Instead of hurling yourself against roadblocks that don't move, choose to see them for what they really are: challenges you can interact with.

A challenge is something we can meet: It calls for action and response. A challenge implies the possibility of growth and change, and that's exactly what it's for. It gives us something to improvise with. This viewpoint creates a positive frame for the unexpected that inspires creative thinking instead of hand-wringing.

Your challenges might be momentary but unavoidable (e.g., an important appointment) or emotional (you feel guilty that you're doing too much for yourself and not enough for your partner). What-ever they are, they'll probably be back, if not in exactly the same guise. Responding to each challenge mindfully, without added angst, pro-vides valuable information about the sorts of things that can get in the way of maintaining your physical activity and how you can deal with them now and in the future. It also helps you develop negotia-tion tools you'll use again and again (with increasing ease) to sustain a physically active life.

As I say to my clients at the end of a session: I wish you many chal-lenges!

Negotiation Strategy #4: Bring Friends and Family On Board

Whenever we change the way we do things, it affects other people. The pushback you get from others may be one of the most difficult chal-lenges you face when you begin putting self-care at the top of the list.

Your new priority may be exciting for you, but family and friends are used to you acting in a certain way. They will likely be surprised and possibly even confused or hurt by some of your new choices. You will need to help the important people in your life understand and accept that taking care of yourself through physical activity has become a new priority for you, and why. Don't just hit them over the head with change and expect them to like it; bring those who will be most affected gently but firmly into your planning.

Once you have decided what you need to do, spread the word. Communicate your self-care needs and physical activity plans and openly discuss them and negotiate with the important people in your life:

» Let them know that physical activity is now going to be a priority for you. Explain that you know it will enhance your well-being and health and give you more energy for all the other things and people in your life, like them.

» Discuss how your new activities might change your schedule. (For example, you normally make breakfast for your family every morning, but now you would like to take a walk before work three days a week. Can your family take responsibility for getting their own breakfast?)

» Talk about what this will mean for the way you usually do things. (On Saturdays, you usually drive your fifteen-year-old daughter to her friend's house a mile away. Let her know that you'd be happy to walk with her there, or she can take the bus that picks her up at the corner.)

» Ask for support and delegate responsibilities. You may get some grumbles, but you may also be surprised by how easily friends and family agree to pick up the slack.

» Tell everyone that you plan to bring physical activity into your whole life. Then make it social and fun and create a culture of

COMMUNICATION PLANNING CHART

What kinds of messages do you need to communicate to friends and family (and yourself) regarding your intention to integrate regular self-care and physical activity into your life? Take some time to think these through before you begin sharing your plans in earnest.

PERSON I NEED TO COMMUNICATE WITH	MESSAGE I WANT TO SEND
Partner	*Honey, I wanted to let you know that I need to take better care of myself. I feel depleted all the time and I want to change this. I decided that I am going to need help from you and the kids to make dinner two nights a week, so I have more time to exercise and we can still eat together.*
Children	*I know you are used to me driving you every Sunday to your friend's house, so I wanted to let you know that I won't be able to do that anymore. I've decided that I need to take better care of myself and have decided to spend a couple of hours every Sunday at the gym. I am happy to give you bus money to get there. Or maybe you want to come with me?*
Friend	*I know we have a standing date to meet for drinks after work on Tuesday, but I wanted to let you know that we'll need to shift that date. I've decided to start taking better care of myself, and part of that looks like it will include getting to the gym after work on Tuesdays and Thursdays to catch a weight class. Do you think Monday or Wednesday will work, or do you want to join me at the gym on Tuesdays?*
Someone else	

movement and well-being wherever you spend time. (For example, ask friends if they would like to make a regular walking date with you, ask your children to ride bikes with you, and ask your partner to hike in a nearby recreation area.) Explore recreational activities and outlets in your community and see what they have to offer. Being active is actually a wonderful way to have fun and spend quality time with friends and loved ones. Help physical activity become an elixir of life for everyone you care about so they can use it to build better lives, too.

Negotiation Strategy #5: Use If-Then Planning

Have you ever had solid intentions only to have them collapse in the face of an unforeseen (but foreseeable) occurrence that you were not prepared to deal with? In life, we can always expect the unexpected. That's why we take out insurance policies. It feels good to know you have something in your back pocket—just in case you need it. The very best insurance policy for making sure you get these valuable experiences from being active is *if-then planning*, the specific backup plan and alternatives you make to overcome the challenges that will certainly arise to your plans.

Simply put, you decide that *if* challenge A occurs, *then* you'll do X, Y, or Z. Once you've got your if-then response, you can pull it out if you need it. Research supports the effectiveness of if-then planning—also called *implementation intentions*—in helping people adopt new behaviors.[8] Implementation intentions offer an effective, low-cost intervention that everyone can do by themselves to change behavior.

Here's a look at how if-then planning works: Sam and Cindy both enrolled in their company's free smoking cessation program, where they were asked to develop if-then plans to help them be more prepared for challenges to quitting. They would determine which situations would most tempt them to smoke and come up with some concrete actions they could take to avoid smoking if those specific situations arose.

Sam identified his "if" situation as the moment after work when he was approached by coworkers to smoke a cigarette with them. His "then" plan was to try to avoid this tempting situation, and if that didn't work, he planned to decline and drive to a nearby park to take a brief walk that would give him similar relaxation benefits to those he got from smoking. Cindy's "if" situation was one of her friends offering her a cigarette when they were hanging out on Saturday night even though they knew she was trying to quit. Her "then" plan was to always carry a pack of gum so instead of just refusing, she could also reach for a stick of gum and satisfy the need to have something in her mouth while being social.

Both Sam and Cindy were surprised to find how empowered they felt just having their Strategies in place. When these challenging situations arose, they were prepared and able to choose their alternative plans without too much trouble. If-then planning changes you from being *reactive* (simply reacting to every challenge without foresight, increasing the likelihood that the challenges will prevail) to being responsive and *proactive* (taking responsibility for protecting your priorities with concrete Strategies you've thought about ahead of time). If-then plans are thought to work because they link a challenging situation with your desired plans ahead of time. This doesn't just give you a plan "in theory." It actually makes your responses more automatic by creating a plan in your mind ahead of time so you actually need less self-control to implement it.[9]

Rather than be bullied by your challenges, teach yourself how to prevent them or even interact with them creatively in the moment. Even if the situation doesn't work the first time, you can genuinely learn from everything that goes awry and apply that learning to develop your future if-then plans. It's very easy. Here's how to do it:

1. *Identify your "if."* Consider the time of day, the people around you, and the general context for your planned physical activity. Given what you know about those things, what challenge is likely to arise when it's time for you to go? Is it a last-minute

request from your boss, your child requesting a snack, or simply your own feeling that you can't stop working? Whatever the specific challenge is, note it. (Remember, one challenge that frequently gets in the way is our belief that we should spend our limited time on taking care of business or other people instead of fueling ourselves. If this is your challenge, note it.)

2. *Figure out your "then."* For each "if," identify one to three Strategies you can use to negotiate the challenge.

3. *Go further.* How might you even prevent this "if" situation from happening in the first place?

See the if-then planning tool below to guide you.

YOUR IF-THEN PLANNING TOOL

IF THIS HAPPENS ...	THEN I WILL ...	HOW CAN I PREVENT THIS FROM HAPPENING IN THE FUTURE?
If I feel too tired after work to go to the gym ...	*Then I will check in with my body and see what type of movement I am up to doing.*	*I can go to sleep earlier the night before or take a walk at lunch instead of waiting until the end of the day.*

Phase 2: Negotiation in Action

Planning is time out; life is all in. The best plans are inevitably moving targets. Negotiation Strategies help you adjust as challenges arise, so that you can improvise in the moment and learn to be flexible about your plans.

You build confidence and negotiation skills by actually negotiating your activities and your other life tasks day by day. A little practice goes a long way. You can learn these techniques on the fly, and you can even practice them with people you trust. Repetition brings results.

Negotiation Strategy #6: Dance with Your Challenges— Be Flexible and Improvise

You plan to go to the gym for forty minutes on Monday after work, and you've been looking forward to it all day. But at 5 p.m., just as you're about to leave, your boss calls you into his office and gives you an urgent assignment that's due in two days. You know you can get the work done in time, but talking with your boss has left you with only twenty minutes for your workout, not the forty you need. Now what are you supposed to do? You leave work fuming about your wrecked plans.

But then you realize that you have a couple of other choices:

» You *still* have twenty minutes that you can use to do something else, like walk over to the park a few blocks away before you drive home.

» You can go home now, jog around the neighborhood before dinner, and do your gym workout tomorrow instead.

Unless you are someone who thrives from and has the luxury of an inflexible schedule, if your approach to physical movement isn't flexible, your physical activity plans will lose out every time the unexpected happens. Life is not a series of either-or choices. We always have alternatives; we just have to mindfully look for them. Being willing to be flexible about your plans, improvise, and think creatively about your options is not only helpful—it's crucial. I like to call this "dancing with your challenges," because that's how it feels. Being adaptable is really a wonderful way to tune in to the opportunities all around us and enjoy moving with them. We can't change the nature of life itself, but we *can* change our expectations about what we can really do.

Our culture teaches us that we can do anything we set our minds to, which generally drives us to always try to impose our goals and ideas on life, in service of achieving our "perfect" plan. When we don't succeed, even because of forces outside our control, we think we've "failed." This mindset really prevents us from sustaining physical activity throughout the ups and downs of life. In contrast, improvisation teaches us to "step into the world" that presents itself in the moment. Giving ourselves Permission to improvise, to allow ourselves to be genuinely curious about the opportunities in whatever context we find ourselves, generates positive emotions that broaden our thinking to more creative responses and alternative solutions.

Negotiation Strategy #7: Hesitate Before You Respond to a Request

When people ask you to do something for them, do you often automatically say yes, even when it interferes with your plans to be physically active? Unless the request is truly urgent, hesitating—which allows you some time to really assess whether you can and want to fulfill a request (based on your physical activity and self-care needs and plans)—is an incredibly useful tool for your negotiation toolbox.

We are often taught that we should learn how to say "no" to requests, so that we can take better care of our own needs. But I believe that the better Strategy is to hesitate, take some space for yourself, and not give a definitive answer until you have a chance to really evaluate whether it's good for you to say yes to the request or not. Then, regardless of whether your answer is yes or no, it will be the right answer for you.

I learned this Strategy from my friend Carol. In fact, it was sage advice that her corporate executive dad gave her before she started her first job out of college. Here's the Strategy:

1. Don't respond to requests immediately (unless they are clearly urgent or essential). Take time to assess your priorities and daily goals and compare them to what has been asked of you: Do you really want to swap the time you had put aside for your physical activity to commit to someone else's needs? Is this request as important as your own revitalization? (This is context-specific so the answer might vary depending on the given day.)

2. Unless the request is urgent, it's okay to gently put the responsibility on the person who is asking for something by requesting that she follow up with you in some way (via email, phone, etc.) so that you can check your calendar or plans.

3. If she doesn't follow up with you, you are off the hook.

4. If she does follow up and your answer is that you can't do it:

   • You do not need to justify with specifics about why you can't do it (unless you really have to).

   • You can sandwich your no with positives. Say, "I wish I could do this for you. But unfortunately, I already have plans I can't change for that time. I hope you find someone else and don't hesitate to ask me again" (if you mean that).

5. If she does follow up with you and your answer is that you can do it, feel good about helping out. Just make sure that you continue to assess your needs with future requests that interfere with your time for self-care.

Negotiation Strategy #8: Listen to Your Body's Messages

We spend so much time logically thinking through what we should do next, making decisions based on expedience, and carrying out our plans. Even when you've committed to making lifelong self-care your goal, it can be hard to let go of the impulse to "do the right thing"—which in this case can seem like doing the exact workout you planned, no matter what. But it's our body's messages that we need to start following.

My client Tanesha, a computer scientist, had had a hard week, dealing with a number of problems at work and two sick children at home whose needs contributed to several sleepless nights. By Friday, she was emotionally and physically exhausted, but she still felt like she should do her full routine at the gym as she'd planned. Luckily, the week before we'd talked about the idea of checking in with her body's messages about how to exercise when she found herself uncertain at the point of decision. So instead of just following her habitual "just do it" mentality, she paused and gave herself time to think.

"Okay, Tanesha," she thought, "just change your clothes, drive to the gym, and work out." She heard the usual voice in her head saying, "Come on, you can do this! Push through." She gritted her teeth. Just thinking about the intense workout was giving her a headache, and she made a conscious effort to unclench her jaw.

"Fine," she thought at first. "I won't do anything. No way I'll make it through my whole routine anyway. I'll just chill on the couch." That was actually pretty appealing. Her muscles were starting to relax on the spot at the prospect of not having to work out hard. But she also felt her shoulders sag with disappointment. Was she copping out? She thought, "I might not be up for my usual workout, but I can do *something*."

Tanesha decided to check in with her body more directly. When we'd discussed doing this in the office, she hadn't sounded too convinced. But at this point, she was ready to give it a try. She shut the door to her office and made sure no one could hear her, and then she began to say in a cheery tone, "Hello body! I know you're wiped out. I know that pushing you hard after all we've been through this week wouldn't be kind to you at all. It wouldn't respect how hard you've worked for me, and it wouldn't respect what you are telling me right now. But you know, and I know, that moving *does* make you feel good and even gives you energy. And we need that. So do you think moving just a little might feel good to do now?" And then, against all her instincts, she waited and listened for a response. She didn't hear any voice, but her instincts told her all she needed to know. Before she knew it, she was out of her chair, out the door, and heading out for a brief ten-minute walk before getting in her car and driving home. Her ten-minute walk turned into a twenty-minute walk. She still felt tired, but she also felt renewed and proud of herself for making the effort to check in with her body on the decision and listen to what it needed at that moment.

Forcing our bodies to do something they're not up for sends the message "chore." This is a pure example of classic conditioning. We do something, experience an effect, and then develop an automatic association between that behavior and the effect. If we force ourselves to exercise in ways that feel bad, we'll likely feel depleted and even stressed from forcing ourselves to do something that deep down we didn't want to do. After we make ourselves exercise in this way a few times, we not only lose our desire to do it but may feel an aversion to it, and decision science suggests that we'll likely choose not to move at all.

Choosing not to do anything can occasionally be the right choice. But once we learn that we have the option, every day, to decide how we want to move, based on how we feel and what else we might be pushing ourselves to accomplish, we are freed to do what we need.

As you get more practiced at tuning in to your body's messages, responding to them with respect and flexibility, you will start to notice which types of physical movement feel pleasurable and good and which types feel draining and bad. Giving yourself Permission to actually listen to your body's cues every day helps you develop a much stronger connection with your core self-care needs and reinforces your motivation to keep moving consistently.

Phase 3: Nonjudgmental Evaluation and Recalibration

Learning is an ongoing process. As you learn ways to let yourself enjoy your physical activities, as you begin looking for and finding new opportunities to move, and as you develop new and creative ways to negotiate your challenges, you learn something else: There's always more you can learn about yourself, what gives you energy and pleasure, and how you can continue to make it an ongoing part of your life. A huge part of this learning process is taking time at the end of every week to nonjudgmentally evaluate how your plans worked out, take note of your experiences and expectations in the real world, see what worked and what didn't work with self-compassion, and recalibrate your plans accordingly.

Negotiation Strategy #9: Learn the Links—Make Physical Activity Relevant and Compelling

One of the most important parts of self-regulation is becoming aware of the feedback you get from the decisions you make. Identifying the links between your movement choice and how you feel in the moment, how you feel afterward, and how it influences what matters most is among the most important feedback systems you can put into place. You can just answer the questions below or review your "What Sustains Us, We Sustain" tree and then answer the questions:

1. After you choose to move, ask yourself:

   * How do I feel?

   * Were any areas of my life improved by this choice?

2. After you choose *not* to move, ask yourself:

- How do I feel?

- Were any areas of my life impacted by this choice?

Simply noticing these links raises your Awareness and gives you a more informed base for your decisions. When you really begin to see the link between, say, an afternoon bike ride and having more patience for your family's needs that evening, and contrast that experience with the connection you noticed between not choosing to do your regular morning physical activity and being less able to concentrate in class that day, you have a more compelling reason to choose physical activity the next time you are at a decision point.

In fact, missing a planned physical activity and also seeing the connections between not moving and how you feel and function is perhaps the strongest motivator for consistency and sustainability that I have identified through my work with clients and informal conversations with people who are regularly active.

I read a personal anecdote in a book that really brings this point home. Ari Weinzweig, cofounder of the internationally renowned Zingerman's Deli in Ann Arbor, Michigan, wrote in his book *A Lapsed Anarchist's Guide to Managing Ourselves* that he didn't really understand how crucial running was for his daily quality of life and functioning, even to his identity, until he got injured and couldn't run.[10] His story resonated with me because the same thing happened to me when I got injured in my twenties and had to stop running while I healed.

Knowing the positive links to your daily life experiences and what matters most from moving gives your physical activity clout. But when you also realize the negative consequences on your day from *not* moving, this information is important feedback to consider and should help you make physical movement a regular priority. Instead of feeling down about missing a planned session, leverage it by identifying the different ways you feel from *not* being active.

Once you bring these links into Awareness, as Jane Brody did (in Chapter 8), they become an even more potent motivator.

Negotiation Strategy #10: Evaluate and Recalibrate with Compassionate Nonjudgment

No one wants to be called names, so why do we so often subject ourselves to name-calling? *I am so lazy. Why did I skip my class—again? Why do I even think I can do this?* When you read those self-judgments, how do you feel? Do they motivate you to be the best you can be? I didn't think so.

Reviewing your week with Awareness, nonjudgment, and self-compassion allows you to celebrate your successes and shows you where you might want to make an adjustment. Remember, you are not aiming for "perfect scores" here; you are embarked on a learning process to become more mindful of what gets in your way so you can become skilled in preventing and overcoming these challenges. There is no failure in this process. Everything that happens or doesn't happen accumulates over time like data from a big experiment you are doing to figure something out. There is no need for judgment because whatever happened is material for you to learn from for the future. Still, not judging this process and letting go of criticizing ourselves when we are used to viewing ourselves as "falling short" is hard to change after so many years of thinking this way.

Self-criticisms are effective and virtually immediate *de*-motivators. Criticizing ourselves when we fail to meet our plans or a standard in some way is just about the worst way for us to motivate ourselves to improve and do better next time. So it should not come as a shock that self-compassion—going easy on ourselves when we haven't conformed to our highest expectations—is positively linked with motivation and well-being in research on health behaviors such as exercise.[11]

Kristen Neff, educational psychologist and author of *Self-Compassion*, has researched self-compassion and written about it extensively.[12] Her research, along with that of others studying self-compassion, suggests that when people become more self-compassionate, their motivation is also enhanced. Self-compassionate people don't have their motivation derailed when they make choices that they later regret. Instead, they address themselves with kindness and understanding, which helps them make note of and learn from their mistakes and then move on without the need for motivation-sapping shame or criticism.[13]

That's right—being kind to yourself instead of critical is a more strategic approach. Individuals who are hard on themselves when it comes to their exercise and self-care put their self-care practices at great risk. Neff's pioneering research on self-compassion has important implications for how we think about things when they go wrong. Monitoring your own self-criticisms, catching yourself, and noticing them with nonjudgment and self-compassion is one of the best ways to stay motivated as you move toward the next choice at hand.

After I read Neff's book, I started using self-compassion in all areas of my life and have found it to be a very powerful way to reduce suffering and negative emotions, fostering kindness instead of cruelty to myself in the aftermath of choices I later regretted. My experiences are supported by the growing body of work on self-compassion suggesting that becoming skilled in having an understanding perspective toward ourselves, our bodies, and our setbacks helps us feel better about ourselves and enhances our motivation for creating behavioral sustainability.

So, after evaluating your past week's plan and how everything played out in real life with self-compassion and nonjudgment, how did it go? Did you get what you wanted? Did your negotiation Strategies work? If they did, fantastic. But if your plans and negotiation Strategies didn't work as well as you had hoped, this is your opportunity to think about why they didn't and what you can change. Then you can try something different *next* week. Recalibrating your expectations and plans based on what you learned during this evaluation of your past week is how you learn what you need for lifelong sustainability.

Changing ourselves and our lives is nothing short of challenging. Choose to learn from every part of your week and feel proud of yourself *no matter what*. Learning how to sustain a revitalizing, joyful, physically active life by actually *living* that life builds confidence, resilience, and a deep knowledge of yourself and your self-care needs to fuel what matters most, which will allow you to dance with all of life's challenges with curiosity, flexibility, and joy.

YOUR WEEKLY COMPASSIONATE AND NONJUDGMENTAL EVALUATION AND RECALIBRATION

Now that you've learned helpful ways to evaluate your past week, you can use the tool below when evaluating in real life.

KEY QUESTIONS	EXAMPLES
What was one success you experienced during the past week?	*I reminded myself to get up from my desk and take a walk around the office.*
What (if anything) got in the way of your planned physical activity?	*My friend showed up at work to surprise me at lunchtime, when I meant to walk, and I said yes to having lunch with her without thinking about it.*
How did your priorities influence your ability to claim time for your physical activity this past week?	*It was always on my mind that I should not sit for so long, and I did manage to at least stand up and stretch my legs several times during the workday.*
What did you learn about prioritizing your physical activity over the past week?	*It's not easy, but I can do it if I remember to.*
How did you feel when you gave yourself Permission to be physically active (or when you didn't)?	*When I was too tired to go to the gym, I didn't go. In retrospect, I could have done something less intense, and will try this next time.*

KEY QUESTIONS	EXAMPLES
How did you feel during and after you participated in physical activity this week? Did it deliver the primary exercise you hoped for?	*I felt energized while I was doing it, in a much better mood than usual after I finished, just as I had hoped I would.*
How did being physically active *take away* from your responsibilities and other people this week?	*I really didn't impose my needs too much on others this week, but maybe next week I'll talk to my partner about having dinner a half-hour later so I can ride my bike after work.*
How did being physically active *benefit* your responsibilities and other people this week?	*Everyone was happy that I was in a better mood.*
Did you choose to fulfill someone else's needs over your own this week? If so, do you know why?	*I had lunch with my friend instead of walking, probably because I always defer to her.*
Did you ever feel selfish during the past week? If so, when? Why do you think you felt that way?	*I felt selfish when I found that I was resenting my friend for making me miss my walk, even though I hadn't seen her in a long time.*
Did you give yourself self-compassion instead of criticism when you made a choice you realized was not the right one?	*After I quickly agreed to have lunch with my friend instead of take my walk, I wanted to kick myself. But then I remembered that being self-compassionate was a better route and it quickly helped me transcend my negativity in the moment. I still have to stop saying yes without thinking, but I realize it's a learning process and I'll give myself time.*
If you could relive the past week (with the same circumstances that occurred), what would you do differently to better take care of yourself or fit in fitness?	*I would remember to bring my comfortable shoes to work so that I would be more likely to take more walking breaks and maybe climb the stairs or go outside.*

The Takeaways

- You negotiate all day long in every context of your life. Self-regulation and negotiation are the lynchpin of lifelong fitness and behavioral sustainability. When your behavior aims to achieve something meaningful, you want to protect it from its challenges.

- Become a skilled self-care negotiator. When you decide to learn negotiation Strategies, you take the reins.

- Negotiation Strategy #1 is to give physical activity clout. Understand the specific value that movement brings to your daily life, giving it influence—or clout—within the dynamics of all of your other daily roles and goals.

- Negotiation Strategy #2 is to plan the logistical issues for the upcoming week. This part of the planning process deals with pragmatic questions: What type of physical activities will help you realize the benefits you want? When will you do them? For how long? Where?

- Negotiation Strategy #3 is to decide to confront challenges, not roadblocks. Responding to each challenge mindfully, without added angst, provides valuable information about the sorts of things that can get in the way of maintaining your physical activity and how you can deal with them now and in the future.

- Negotiation Strategy #4 is to bring friends and family on board. Being active is a wonderful way to have fun and spend quality time with friends and loved ones.

- Negotiation Strategy #5 is to use if-then planning. This is the very best insurance policy for making sure you get the valuable experiences you want from being active. The specific back-up plan and alternatives you make helps you to overcome the challenges that will arise to your plans.

- Negotiation Strategy #6 is to dance with your challenges, be flexible, and improvise. Being willing to be flexible, improvise, and think creatively about your options will help you develop more effective Strategies and is key for sustaining a physically active life.

- Negotiation Strategy #7 is to hesitate before you respond to a request. Allow yourself some time to really assess whether you can and want to fulfill any given request, based on your needs and plans.

- Negotiation Strategy #8 is to listen to your body's messages. Forcing your body to do something it's not up for sends the message "chore." If you force yourself to exercise in ways that feel bad, you'll likely choose not to move at all.

- Negotiation Strategy #9 is to learn the links between being physically active and the rest of your day. Identify the links between not moving and moving and how you feel. Notice how your choices influence your physical and mental states and how that further influences what matters most.

- Negotiation Strategy #10 is to evaluate and recalibrate with compassion and nonjudgment. Reviewing your week this way allows you to celebrate your successes and become more mindful of what gets in your way so you can become skilled in preventing and overcoming these challenges.

Epilogue

Changing Your Beliefs, Changing Your Behavior, Changing Your Life

Your beliefs become your thoughts,
Your thoughts become your words,
Your words become your actions,
Your actions become your habits,
Your habits become your values,
Your values become your destiny.

—MAHATMA GANDHI

OUR BELIEFS ARE LIKE THE AIR WE BREATHE: INVISIBLE. YET, LIKE AIR, they are essential. Our beliefs mold our experience and actions, inform our judgments, and are central to who we are.[1] Our beliefs actually seed our goals, choices, and behavior. So if we want to change our behavior, we must start by changing our beliefs about what's possible.

I'd like to share this story from my client Stephanie. She wrote to me serendipitously, just as I was finishing the last chapter of *No Sweat*, to share her incredible journey with being physically active. Her journey shows the ways in which physical activity can transform from a chore into a gift, eventually metamorphosing into something completely different—essential fuel for the resilience we need when life takes unexpected turns.

Stephanie's Story: MAPS in Real Life

When I started working with you, I was coming off of over a decade of exercising for all the wrong reasons. Throughout my teens and twenties, I believed that "working out" meant "running fast for at least forty-five minutes, four to six days a week." That's what my husband liked to do, that's what many of my thinner friends did—and it's what I'd managed to do for about two years, even when it meant completing a half-marathon with food poisoning or running on a stress fracture. The foot injury finally derailed my running ambitions, and I was secretly grateful—I had never looked forward to running. It was simply a chore to cram into my already busy life, so I could stay my high school size forever. But without running, of course, the weight started to creep on. And I began to feel like I had "failed" at exercise. I got stuck in a vicious cycle, dragging myself back out there to try to lose the weight, then getting frustrated and giving up.

Then I started your program. Through our work together, I learned to rethink my definition of "working out." I used to believe that I had to be a runner to "succeed" at exercise. Now I believe that gardening can be a workout. Yoga can be a workout. Hiking or even just walking around my neighborhood can be a workout. You taught me to look beyond the scale, to find all the other ways that physical activity could benefit my life. I began to see how prioritizing time to exercise actually made it easier to keep my stress level in check, to fit in quality time with my husband and friends, and even to feel better about my body. In truth, the scale didn't budge. But I felt stronger and more capable when I realized that being able to do a headstand in yoga, or mulch all my flower beds by myself, was equally as valid as being able to run an eight-minute mile.

By the time I finished your six-week program, I felt invigorated by my new relationship with movement. I had a whole long list of the kinds of physical activity I enjoyed and a lot of Strategies and tools for helping me make the time to do it. But there was a part of me that was still skeptical—I felt like I'd made these big changes, but I wasn't sure how well I would sustain them without a weekly phone call with you to keep me on track. I was also pregnant for the first time and wondering how on earth I would keep fitness in my life once I became a new mom.

Then my daughter was born with complex congenital heart defects. Forget everything I'd imagined about fitting in Mommy & Me stroller workouts or taking long walks with my baby snuggled in the Ergo baby carrier. My first year of parenthood involved spending almost eighty days living in a hospital PICU while my daughter fought for her life, undergoing seven surgical procedures (including two open heart operations) before she was nine months old.

Under those circumstances, I hope even the most diehard exercise fanatics would forgive themselves for never getting to the gym. As important as it is to prioritize exercise when we can (for all those amazing benefits), there are simply times in life when it cannot and should not matter as much. So there were many days when I barely moved out of the chair by my daughter's hospital crib. But more often, especially once we were out of the initial emergency situation and into the grind of undergoing and recovering from repeated surgeries, I came to understand how physical movement can support and sustain us through our darkest times.

In fact, the year I had my daughter and we went through this horrific medical journey is also the year I discovered my passion for swimming. I had taken lessons during the long, hot summer of my pregnancy and fell in love with the water. But to be honest, when I initially dragged myself to the pool at my gym a few weeks after my daughter's first heart surgery, it was with some ambivalence; I was anxious about being away from her and convinced that I just "didn't have time" to "worry about working out." As I drove there, my mind was an endless loop of worry about my daughter, about the work projects I was returning to, about whether we'd ever sleep through the night again.

Then I got in the water and, as I pushed forward into my first lap, my mind cleared. There were a few other swimmers in the pool, but when I opened my eyes underwater, I mostly just saw blue. When I came up for air, I faced the gym's windows so I mostly saw sun. I repeated blue, sun, blue, sun for lap after lap. Even as my heart rate sped up, I felt like I could breathe more freely than I had since the day my daughter was diagnosed.

Swimming let me release all of the fear, worry, and stress. It became my escape and my solace during this impossible year. It's made me stronger, physically and mentally, besides being just downright fun—something that I was otherwise definitely not having very often under these circumstances. And in my case, movement begets movement. While I can't make the time to swim every day, now I believe that physical activity helps and heals me. Because of that core belief, when I can't make time to swim, I find other ways to fit in smaller workouts. I even keep a series of yoga videos downloaded on my iPhone so when we're in the hospital with my daughter, I can grab ten minutes here and there to stretch, strengthen, and center myself. I don't beat myself up when it doesn't happen, because I now believe that the actual workout on any given day doesn't really matter.

It isn't about how fast you run or how far you swim, though I do still find those small goals fun and motivating. It's about the big picture: Movement is something I'll always want and return to in the course of my life. It's not a chore or an unattainable weight loss goal; it's a part of who I am.

Stephanie's poignant story illustrates MAPS in action in the real world: Learning new information about being physically active, especially why and how we do it, combined with interacting with these new beliefs through new experiences and giving ourselves Permission to take care of ourselves within the realities of our lives, join together and transform our understanding of the true value of physical movement in our complex, dynamic lives.

The Learning Process Never Ends

Examining what we have learned to believe about physical activity, about our priorities, and about taking care of ourselves, as Stephanie did, is the place to start. My MAPS process reflects Paulo Freire's method of beginning with what he calls *conscientization*,[2] a process that lets each of us critically reflect on what we have learned to believe about exercising within society. As Stephanie discovered, gaining Awareness of the Meaning exercise had for her (especially why and how she was supposed to be doing it), and comparing these beliefs to the unsatisfying outcomes she was getting, actually liberated her from those limiting beliefs. That realization allowed her to take responsibility for her Meaning. She formed a new personalized and empowering relationship with being physically active, one that aimed to reduce her stress and fit in quality time with her husband and friends.

None of this would have happened if Stephanie had not been willing to look at the role that her own beliefs about exercising had played in her dislike of exercise and her unwillingness to prioritize it. The changes that grew out of her new understanding led her to believe more in herself, be more self-compassionate, and even feel better about her body (whether or not there were any changes on the scale). They also created a new space to give herself Permission to prioritize movement and use Strategies that enabled her to maintain movement beyond the short time that she worked with me.

As Freire suggests, the process never ends. Our physical activity and self-care needs are always embedded within the current realities of our lives, however challenging they may be. As Stephanie's life became dark with worry and stress about her ill newborn, this created a new context for her physical activity. At first, she could find no space in this context for movement because she couldn't bear to leave her daughter's side. But after her daughter's health became less critical, Stephanie knew she had to return to her own self-care so she could keep up the hard work of caring for her daughter. Stephanie's beliefs about and Meaning for exercise shifted once again as swimming became her solace and escape, an ally that gave her the resilience and energy she needed to tend to her daughter during that heart-wrenching year.

The interplay between physical movement and her life experiences further deepened Stephanie's Meaning of physical movement. She now recognized movement as a core part of who she is. Stephanie originally came to me to help her change her behavior, but that wasn't really what she needed. Instead of behavior change per se, she needed to change her beliefs so she could integrate the *value of* physical activity within her sense of self and life.[3] When our daily choices and actions align with our core selves, it energizes our day and helps us with being who we are; it gives us *well-being*. And we are continually fueled for what matters most.

Your Journey Continues

Feel free to review MAPS and revisit all of your answers to the *It's Your Move* questions to critically evaluate whether they have changed in any way and what new experiences you need to have in order to deepen what you know. Remember, learning to sustain a physically active life requires that you investigate your beliefs about physical activity and self-care through having new experiences and gaining new knowledge within the realities of your life. It's a dynamic, ongoing process in which you reflect on what you are learning and change your beliefs about physical activity, self-care, and even yourself as you see fit. This is your journey, you're in the driver's seat, and now you've got your MAPS.

I hope that *No Sweat* has helped you understand the hidden reasons you've had difficulty sustaining a physically active life and prioritizing your self-care, and that you now are beginning to understand what you can do in order to create a physically active life that revitalizes you to live your life joyfully and in meaningful ways. Unless you have a medical need that prevents you from following this advice, I encourage you to work on learning how to sustain a physically active life for at least three months, if not two years, before starting another major behavior change process.

Physical activity is not only an elixir of life—it's the foundation of a lifetime of fitness, health, meaning, and well-being. It's something that you can lean on in times of need. You've got the rest of your life to be active. Why not take enough time to make sure you learn how to enjoy it and to stick with it throughout its inevitable ups and downs? And here's a secret: Once you feel comfortable and confident that you've internalized the value of consistent physical movement, you can use my MAPS system to adopt any other behavior into your life.

A behavior is meaningful only when it effectively delivers an outcome that we highly value.[4] I hope you are ready to discover how physical activity can feel great and become deeply meaningful to you and your life, and then choose to move in ways that deliver those valued outcomes. Remember, you're on a journey, not aiming at a bull's-eye. Let go of ideas of perfection and enjoy finding your way, rough spots and all.

And above all else, remember: What sustains us, we sustain.

Endnotes

Chapter 1. It's Not About the Sweat

1. In 2012, ABC News reported that the annual revenue of the U.S. weight-loss industry was $20 billion and that 108 million people in the United States were on diets. "100 Million Dieters; $20 Billion: The Weight-Loss Industry By the Numbers." http://abcnews.go.com/Health/100-million-dieters-20-billion-weight-loss-industry/story?id=16297197. Accessed July 26, 2014.

2. Michelle Segar, Victor Katch, and Randy Roth, "The Effects of Aerobic Exercise on Self-Esteem and Depressive and Anxiety Symptoms Among Breast Cancer Survivors," *Oncology Nursing Forum* 25, 1998, 107–113.

3. Michelle Segar, Toby Jayaratne, Jennifer Hanlon, and Caroline R. Richardson, "Fitting Fitness into Women's Lives: Effects of a Gender-Tailored Physical Activity Intervention," *Women's Health Issues* 12(6), November–December 2002, 338–347.

4. Howard Leventhal, Ian Brissette, and Elaine A. Leventhal, "The Common-Sense Model of Self-Regulation of Health and Illness," in *The Self-Regulation of Health and Illness Behaviour*, edited by Linda D. Cameron and Howard Leventhal (New York: Routledge, 2003), 42–65.

5. Julius Kuhl, "A Functional-Design Approach to Motivation and Self-Regulation: The Dynamics of Personality Systems Interactions," in *Handbook of Self-Regulation*, edited by Monique Boekaerts, Paul R. Pintrich, and Moshe Zeidner (Burlington, Mass.: Elsevier Academic Press, 2000), 111–169.

6. Ian McGregor and Brian R. Little, "Personal Projects, Happiness, and Meaning: On Doing Well and Being Yourself," *Journal of Personality and Social Psychology* 74(2), February 1998, 494–512.

7. Brian R. Little, Susan D. Phillips, and Katariina Salmela-Aro, eds., *Personal Project Pursuit: Goals, Action, and Human Flourishing* (Mahwah, N.J.: Lawrence Erlbaum Associates, 2007); Brian R. Little, *Me, Myself, and Us: The Science of Personality and the Art of Well-Being* (New York: Public Affairs, 2014).

Chapter 2. Escaping the Vicious Cycle of Failure

1. Statistic Brain, "Gym Membership Statistics." http://www.statisticbrain.com/gym-membership-statistics/. Accessed July 27, 2014.

2. Benjamin K. Bergen, *Louder Than Words: The New Science of How the Mind Makes Meaning* (New York: Basic Books, 2012), 3.

3. Daniel Cervone, William G. Shadel, Ronald E. Smith, and Marina Fiori, "Self-Regulation: Reminders and Suggestions from Personality Science," *Applied Psychology* 55(3), July 2006, 333–385; Jacquelynne Eccles, "Who Am I and What Am I Going to Do With My Life?: Personal and Collective Identities as Motivators of Action," *Educational Psychologist* 44(2), 2009, 78–89.

4. Donna Spruijt-Metz, *Adolescence, Affect and Health* (East Sussex, U.K.: Psychology Press, 1999); Howard Leventhal, Ian Brissette, and Elaine A. Leventhal, "The Common-Sense Model of Self-Regulation of Health and Illness," in *The Self-Regulation of Health and Illness Behaviour*, edited by Linda D. Cameron and Howard Leventhal (New York: Routledge, 2003), 42–65.

5. Spruijt-Metz, *Adolescence*.

6. Michelle L. Segar, Jacquelynne S. Eccles, and Caroline R. Richardson, "Rebranding Exercise: Closing the Gap Between Values and Behavior," *International Journal of Behavioral Nutrition and Physical Activity* 8(94), 2011, 1–4.

7. Rebecca Lawton, Mark Conner, and Rosemary McEachan, "Desire or Reason: Predicting Health Behaviors from Affective and Cognitive Attitudes," *Health Psychology* 28(1), January 2009, 56–65; Mario Keer, Bas van den Putte, and Peter Neijens, "The Role of Affect and Cognition in Health Decision Making," *British Journal of Social Psychology* 49(1), March 2010, 143–153; Mark Conner, Ryan E. Rhodes, Ben Morris, Rosemary McEachan, and Rebecca Lawton, "Changing Exercise Through Targeting Affective or Cognitive Attitudes," *Psychology & Health* 26(2), 2011, 133–149.

8. Nico H. Frijda, *The Emotions* (Cambridge, U.K.: Cambridge University Press, 1986).

9. Charles S. Carver and Michael F. Scheier, *On the Self-Regulation of Behavior* (Cambridge, U.K.: Cambridge University Press, 1998).

10. Kathleen D. Vohs and Todd F. Heatherton, "Self-Regulatory Failure: A Resource-Depletion Approach," *Psychological Science* 11(3), May 2000, 249–254.

11. Dylan D. Wagner, Myra Altman, Rebecca G. Boswell, William M. Kelley, and Todd F. Heatherton, "Self-Regulatory Depletion Enhances Neural Responses to Rewards and Impairs Top-Down Control," *Psychological Science* 24(11), November 2013, 2262–2271.

12. Larissa K. Barber and David C. Munz, "Consistent-Sufficient Sleep Predicts Improvements in Self-Regulatory Performance and Psychological Strain," *Stress and Health* 27(4), October 2011, 314–324.

13. Mark Muraven, Roy F. Baumeister, and Dianne M. Tice, "Longitudinal Improvement of Self-Regulation Through Practice: Building Self-Control Strength Through Repeated Exercise," *Journal of Social Psychology* 139(4), August 1999, 446–457.

Chapter 3. Motivation from the Inside Out

1. Daniel Cervone, William G. Shadel, Ronald E. Smith, and Marina Fiori, "Self-Regulation: Reminders and Suggestions from Personality Science," *Applied Psychology* 55(3), July 2006, 333–385.

2. Richard S. Lazarus, "Cognition and Motivation in Emotion," *American Psychologist* 46(4), April 1991, 352–367.

3. Ibid.

4. Howard Leventhal, Ian Brissette, and Elaine A. Leventhal, "The Common-Sense Model of Self-Regulation of Health and Illness," in *The Self-Regulation of Health and Illness Behaviour*, edited by Linda D. Cameron and Howard Leventhal (New York: Routledge, 2003), 43–65.

5. Richard M. Ryan and Edward L. Deci, "Self-Determination Theory and the Facilitation of Intrinsic Motivation, Social Development, and Well-Being," *American Psychologist* 55(1), January 2000, 68–78. Dan H. Pink, *Drive: The Surprising Truth About What Motivates Us* (New York: Riverhead Books, 2011).

6. Pedro J. Teixeira, Eliana V. Carraca, David Markland, Marlene N. Silva, and Richard M. Ryan, "Exercise, Physical Activity, and Self-Determination Theory: A Systematic Review," *International Journal of Behavioral Nutrition and Physical Activity* 9(78), 2012, 1–30.

7. Juliano Laran and Chris Janiszewski, "Work or Fun?: How Task Construal and Completion Influence Regulatory Behavior," *Journal of Consumer Research* 37, April 2011, 967–983.

8. Charles S. Carver and Michael F. Scheier, *On the Self-Regulation of Behavior* (Cambridge: Cambridge University Press, 1998); Richard P. Bagozzi, Hans Baumgartner, and Rik Pieters, "Goal-Directed Emotions," *Cognition and Emotion* 12(1), 1998, 1–26.

9. Julius Kuhl, "A Functional-Design Approach to Motivation and Self-Regulation: The Dynamics of Personality Systems and Interactions," in *Handbook of Self-Regulation*, edited by Monique Boekaerts, Paul R. Pintrich, and Moshe Zeidner (Burlington, Mass.: Elsevier Academic Press, 2000), 111–169.

10. Charles S. Carver and Michael F. Scheier, "On the Structure of Behavioral Self-Regulation," in *Handbook of Self-Regulation*, edited by Monique Boekaerts, Paul R. Pintrich, and Moshe Zeidner (Burlington, Mass.: Elsevier Academic Press, 2000), 41–84.

11. Maarten Vansteenkiste, Christopher P. Niemiec, and Bart Soenens, "The Development of the Five Mini-Theories of Self-Determination Theory: An Historical Overview, Emerging Trends, and Future Directions," in *The Decade Ahead: Theoretical Perspectives on Motivation and Achievement*, edited by Timothy C. Urdan and Stuart A. Karabenick (Bingley, U.K.: Emerald Group, 2010), 105 165.

12. Michelle L. Segar, Jacquelynne S. Eccles, Stephen C. Peck, and Caroline R. Richardson, "Midlife Women's Physical Activity Goals: Socio-Cultural Influences and Effects on Behavioral Regulation," *Sex Roles* 57(11/12), December 2007, 837–850.

13. Carolina O. C. Werle, Brian Wansink, and Collin R. Payne, "Is it Fun or Exercise?: The Framing of Physical Activity Biases Subsequent Snacking," *Marketing Letters*, 2014, 1–12.

14. Amy Wrzesniewski, Barry Schwartz, Xinagyu Cong, Michael Kane, Audrey Omar, and Thomas Kolditz, "Multiple Types of Motives Don't Multiply the Motivation of West Point Cadets," *Proceedings of the National Academy of Sciences* 111(30), July 29, 2014, 10990–10995.

15. Michal Maimaran and Ayelet Fishbach, "If It's Useful and You Know It, Do You Eat?: Preschoolers Refrain from Instrumental Food," *Journal of Consumer Research* 41(3), October 2014, 642–655.

16. Ying Zhang, Ayelet Fishbach, and Arie W. Kruglanski, "The Dilution Model: How Additional Goals Undermine the Perceived Instrumentality of a Shared Path," *Journal of Personality and Social Psychology* 92(3), March 2007, 389–401.

17. Paul Sparks, Peter R. Harris, and Nina Lockwood, "Predictors and Predictive Effects of Ambivalence," *British Journal of Social Psychology* 43(3), September 2004, 371–383.

Chapter 4. Exorcising Exercise

1. Michelle Segar, Donna Spruijt-Metz, and Susan Nolen-Hoeksema, "Go Figure?: Body-Shaping Motives Are Associated with Decreased Physical Activity Participation Among Midlife Women," *Sex Roles* 55(3/4), February 2006, 175–187.

2. Seymour Epstein and Rosemary Pacini, "Some Basic Issues Regarding Dual-Process Theories from the Perspective of Cognitive-Experimental Self-Theory," in *Dual-Process Theories in Social Psychology*, edited by Shelly Chaiken and Yaacov Trope (New York: Guilford Press, 1999), 462–482; Wilhelm Hofmann, Malte Friese, and Reinout W. Wiers, "Impulsive Versus Reflective Influences on Health Behavior: A Theoretical Framework and Empirical Review," *Health Psychology Review* 2(2), September 2008, 111–137.

3. Richard S. Lazarus, "Cognition and Motivation in Emotion," *American Psychologist* 46(4), April 1991, 352–367; Esther K. Papies and Henk Aarts, "Non-conscious Self-Regulation, or the Automatic Pilot of Human Behavior," in *Handbook of Self-Regulation: Research, Theory, and Applications*, 2nd ed., edited by Kathleen D. Vohs and Roy F. Baumeister (New York: Guilford Press, 2011), 125–142.

4. Reinout W. Wiers, Katrijn Houben, Anne Roefs, Peter de Jong, Wilhelm Hofmann, and Alan W. Stacy, "Implicit Cognition in Health Psychology: Why Common Sense Goes Out the Window," in *Handbook of Implicit Social Cognition: Measurement, Theory, and Applications*, edited by Bertram Gawronski and B. Keith Payne (New York: Guilford Press, 2010), 463–488.

5. Hannah H. Chang and Michel Tuan Pham, "Affect as a Decision-Making System of the Present," *Journal of Consumer Research* 40(1), June 2013, 42–63.

6. Steven J. Petruzzello, "Doing What Feels Good (and Avoiding What Feels Bad)—A Growing Recognition of the Influence of Affect on Exercise Behavior: A Comment on Williams et al.," *Annals of Behavioral Medicine* 44(1), May 2012, 7–9.

7. Panteleimon Ekkekakis, "Redrawing the Model of the Exercising Human in Exercise Prescriptions: From Headless Manikin to a Creature with Feelings!" in *Lifestyle Medicine*, 2nd ed., edited by James M. Rippe (Boca Raton, Fla.: CRC Press, 2013), 1421–1433.

8. Panteleimon Ekkekakis, Gaynor Parfitt, and Steven J. Petruzzello, "The Pleasure and Displeasure People Feel When They Exercise at Different Intensities: Decennial Update and Progress Towards a Tripartite Rationale for Exercise Intensity Prescription," *Sports Medicine* 41(8), 2011, 641–671.

9. Gina Kolata, *Ultimate Fitness: The Quest for Truth about Exercise and Health* (New York: Farrar, Straus, and Giroux, 2003), 4.

10. Ekkekakis, Parfitt and Petruzzello, "The Pleasure and Displeasure."

11. David M. Williams, Shira Dunsiger, Robert Miranda, Chad J. Gwaltney, Jessica A. Emerson, Peter M. Monti, and Alfred F. Parisi, "Recommending Self-Paced Exercise among Overweight and Obese Adults: A Randomized Pilot Study," *Annals of Behavioral Medicine*, 2014.

12. Marlene N. Silva, David Markland, Eliana V. Carraça, Paulo N. Vieira, Silvia R. Coutinho, Claudia S. Minderico, Margarida G. Matos, Luis B. Sardinha, and Pedro J. Teixeira, "Exercise Autonomous Motivation Predicts 3-yr Weight Loss in Women," *Medicine & Science in Sports & Exercise* 43(4), April 2011, 728–737.

Chapter 5. Count Everything and Choose to Move!

1. U.S. Department of Health and Human Services, *Physical Activity and Health: A Report of the Surgeon General* (Atlanta, Ga.: Centers for Disease Control and Prevention, National Center for Chronic Disease Prevention and Health Promotion, 1996).

2. William L. Haskell, I-Min Lee, Russell R. Pate, Kenneth E. Powell, Steven N. Blair, Barry A. Franklin, Caroline A. Macera, Gregory W. Heath, Paul D. Thompson, and Adrian Bauman, "Physical Activity and Public Health: Updated Recommendation for Adults from the American College of Sports Medicine and the American Heart Association," *Circulation* 116(9), August 28, 2007, 1081–1093.

3. Russell R. Pate, Michael Pratt, Steven N. Blair, William L. Haskell, Caroline A. Macera, Claude Bouchard, David Buchner, et al., "Physical Activity and Public Health. A Recommendation from the Centers for Disease Control and Prevention and the American College of Sports Medicine," *Journal of the American Medical Association* 273(5), 1995, 402–407.

4. Janine Clarke and Ian Janssen, "Sporadic and Bouted Physical Activity and the Metabolic Syndrome in Adults," *Medicine & Science in Sports & Exercise* 46(1), January 2014, 76–83; Paul D. Loprinzi and Bradley J. Cardinal, "Association Between Biologic Outcomes and Objectively Measured Physical Activity Accumulated in ≥ 10-Minute Bouts and < 10-Minute Bouts," *American Journal of Health Promotion* 27(3), January–February 2013, 143–151.

5. Thomas Bossmann, Martina Kanning, Susanne Koudela-Hamila, Stefan Hey, and Ulrich Ebner-Priemer, "The Association Between Short Periods of Everyday Life Activities and Affective States: A Replication Study Using Ambulatory Assessment," *Frontiers in Psychology* 4(102), April 15, 2013, 1–7.

6. Marc T. Hamilton, Deborah G. Hamilton, and Theodore W. Zderic, "Role of Low Energy Expenditure and Sitting in Obesity, Metabolic Syndrome, Type 2 Diabetes, and Cardiovascular Disease," *Diabetes* 56(11), November 2007, 2655–2667; Marc T. Hamilton, Deborah G. Hamilton, and Theodore W.

Zderic, "Sedentary Behavior as a Mediator of Type 2 Diabetes," *Medicine and Sport Science* 60, 2014, 11–26.

7. Marc T. Hamilton, Genevieve N. Healy, David W. Dunstan, Theodore W. Zderic, and Neville Owen, "Too Little Exercise and Too Much Sitting: Inactivity Physiology and the Need for New Recommendations on Sedentary Behavior," *Current Cardiovascular Risk Reports* 2(4), July 2008, 292–298.

8. Per Sjögren, Rachel Fisher, Lena Kallings, Ulrika Svenson, Göran Roos, and Mai-Lis Hellénius, "Stand Up for Health—Avoiding Sedentary Behaviour Might Lengthen Your Telomeres: Secondary Outcomes from a Physical Activity RCT in Older People," *British Journal of Sports Medicine* 48(19), 2014, 1407–1409.

9. Gregory W. Heath, J. R. Gavin, J. M. Hinderliter, James M. Hagberg, Susan A. Bloomfield, and John O. Holloszy, "Effects of Exercise and Lack of Exercise on Glucose-Tolerance and Insulin Sensitivity," *Journal of Applied Physiology* 55(2), August 1983, 512–517.

10. Scott J. Strath, Robert G. Holleman, David L. Ronis, Ann M. Swartz, and Caroline R. Richardson, "Objective Physical Activity Accumulation in Bouts and Nonbouts and Relation to Markers of Obesity in US Adults," *Preventing Chronic Disease* 5(4), 2008, 1–11.

11. M. Robin DiMatteo, "Variations in Patients' Adherence to Medical Recommendations: A Quantitative Review of 50 Years of Research," *Medical Care* 42(3), 2004, 200–209.

12. Dan Ariely, *Predictably Irrational: The Hidden Forces That Shape Our Decisions*, rev. ed. (New York: Harper Perennial, 2010).

13. Pierre Chandon and Brian Wansink, "Does Food Marketing Need to Make Us Fat?: A Review and Solutions," *Nutrition Reviews* 70(10), October 2012, 571–593.

14. Michelle Segar, Toby Jayaratne, Jennifer Hanlon, and Caroline R. Richardson, "Fitting Fitness into Women's Lives: Effects of a Gender-Tailored Physical Activity Intervention," *Women's Health Issues* 12(6), November–December 2002, 338–347.

15. Steve Amireault, Gaston Godin, and Lydi-Anne Vezina-Im, "Determinants of Physical Activity Maintenance: A Systematic Review and Meta-Analyses," *Health Psychology Review* 7(1), 2013, 55–91.

16. Deborah Kendzierski, "Exercise Self-Schemata: Cognitive and Behavioral Correlates," *Health Psychology* 9(1), 1990, 69–82; Shaelyn M. Strachan, Jennifer Woodgate, Lawrence R. Brawley, and Adrienne Tse, "The Relationship of Self-Efficacy and Self-Identity to Long-Term Maintenance of Vigorous Physical Activity," *Journal of Applied Biobehavioral Research* 10(2), April 2005, 98–112.

17. Jason Duvall, "Enhancing the Benefits of Outdoor Walking with Cognitive Engagement Strategies," *Journal of Environmental Psychology* 31(1), 2011, 27–35.

Chapter 6. From a Chore to a Gift

1. John J. Ratey and Eric Hagerman, *Spark: The Revolutionary New Science of Exercise and the Brain* (New York: Little, Brown and Company, 2008); Steriani

Elavsky and Edward McAuley, "Physical Activity, Symptoms, Esteem, and Life Satisfaction During Menopause," *Maturitas* 52(3-4), November-December 2005, 374-385; Jaswinder Chahal, Raymond Lee, and Jin Luo, "Loading Dose of Physical Activity Is Related to Muscle Strength and Bone Density in Middle-Aged Women," *Bone* 67, October 2014, 41-45; Francisco Perales, Jose del Pozo-Cruz, Jesus del Pozo-Cruz, and Borja del Pozo-Cruz, "On the Associations Between Physical Activity and Quality of Life: Findings from an Australian Nationally Representative Panel Survey," *Quality of Life Research* 23(7), September 2014, 1921-1933; Jennifer Huberty, Jamie Vener, Yong Gao, Justin L. Matthews, Lynda Ransdell, and Steriani Elavsky, "Developing an Instrument to Measure Physical Activity Related Self-Worth in Women: Rasch Analysis of the Women's Physical Activity Self-Worth Inventory (WPASWI)," *Psychology of Sport and Exercise* 14(1), January 2013, 111-121; Thomas Bossmann, Martina Kanning, Susanne Koudela-Hamila, Stefan Hey, and Ulrich Ebner-Priemer, "The Association Between Short Periods of Everyday Life Activities and Affective States: A Replication Study Using Ambulatory Assessment," *Frontiers in Psychology* 4(102), April 15, 2013, 1-7; Jaclyn P. Maher, Shawna E. Doerksen, Steriani Elavsky, Amanda L. Hyde, Aaron L. Pincus, Nilam Ram, and David E. Conroy, "A Daily Analysis of Physical Activity and Satisfaction with Life in Emerging Adults," *Health Psychology* 32(6), June 2013, 647-656; Kathleen A. Martin Ginis, Heather A. Strong, Shawn M. Arent, Steven R. Bray, and Rebecca L. Bassett-Gunter, "The Effects of Aerobic- Versus Strength-Training on Body Image Among Young Women with Pre-existing Body Image Concerns," *Body Image* 11(3), June 2014, 219-227.

2. Hannah H. Chang and Michel Tuan Pham, "Affect as a Decision-Making System of the Present," *Journal of Consumer Research* 40(1), June 2013, 42-63.

3. Ahmad R. Hariri, Sarah M. Brown, Douglas E. Williamson, Janine D. Flory, Harriet de Wit, and Stephen B. Manuck, "Preference for Immediate Over Delayed Rewards Is Associated with Magnitude of Ventral Striatal Activity," *Journal of Neuroscience* 26(51), December 2006, 13213-13217.

4. Dan Ariely, "Why We Do Things That Aren't in Our Best Interests," http://bigthink.com/videos/why-we-do-things-that-arent-in-our-best-interests.

5. Michelle Segar, Toby Jayaratne, Jennifer Hanlon, and Caroline R. Richardson, "Fitting Fitness into Women's Lives: Effects of a Gender-Tailored Physical Activity Intervention," *Women's Health Issues* 12(6), November-December 2002, 338-347.

6. Kent C. Berridge, Terry E. Robinson, and J. Wayne Aldridge, "Dissecting Components of Reward: 'Liking', 'Wanting', and Learning," *Current Opinions in Pharmacology* 9(1), February 2009, 65-73.

7. Ruud Custers and Henk Arts, "Positive Affect as Implicit Motivator: On the Nonconscious Operation of Behavioral Goals," *Journal of Personality and Social Psychology* 89(2), August 2005, 129-142.

8. Panteleimon Ekkekakis, Gaynor Parfitt, and Steven J. Petruzzello, "The Pleasure and Displeasure People Feel When They Exercise at Different Intensities: Decennial Update and Progress Towards a Tripartite Rationale for Exercise Intensity Prescription," *Sports Medicine* 41(8), 2011, 641-671.

9. Melinda Asztalos, Ilse De Bourdeaudhuij, and Greet Cardon, "The Relation-

ship Between Physical Activity and Mental Health Varies Across Activity Intensity Levels and Dimensions of Mental Health Among Women and Men," *Public Health Nutrition* 13(8), August 2010, 1207–1214.

10. America Walks, http://americawalks.org/; "Every Body Walk! The Campaign to Get America Walking," http://everybodywalk.org/. Accessed September 18, 2014.

11. Surgeon General Announces Call to Action on Walking," http://usa.streetsblog.org/2012/12/05/surgeon-general-announces-call-to-action-on-walking/. Accessed September 18, 2014.

12. Marie Murphy, Alan Nevill, Charlotte Neville, Stuart Biddle, and Adrianne Hardman, "Accumulating Brisk Walking for Fitness, Cardiovascular Risk, and Psychological Health," *Medicine & Science in Sports & Exercise*, 34(9), 2002, 1468–1474; Melissa R. Marselle, Katherine N. Irvine, and Sara L. Warber, "Walking for Well-Being: Are Group Walks in Certain Types of Natural Environments Better for Well-Being than Group Walks in Urban Environments?" *International Journal of Environmental Research and Public Health* 10(11), 2013, 5603–5628; Jong-Hwan Park, Masashi Miyashita, Masaki Takahashi, Noriaki Kawanishi, Harumi Hayashida, Hyun-Shik Kim, Katsuhiko Suzuki, and Yoshio Nakamura, "Low-Volume Walking Program Improves Cardiovascular-Related Health in Older Adults," *Journal of Sports Science and Medicine* 13(3), September 2014, 624–631.

13. Gregory A. Brown, Chad M. Cook, Ryan D. Krueger, and Kate A. Heelan, "Comparison of Energy Expenditure on a Treadmill vs. an Elliptical Device at a Self-Selected Exercise Intensity," *Journal of Strength and Conditioning Research* 24(6), 2010, 1643–1649.

14. Elaine A. Rose and Gaynor Parfitt, "Can the Feeling Scale Be Used to Regulate Exercise Intensity?" *Medicine & Science in Sports & Exercise* 40(10), 2008, 1852–1860.

15. Gretchen Rubin, *The Happiness Project: Or, Why I Spent a Year Trying to Sing in the Morning, Clean My Closets, Fight Right, Read Aristotle, and Generally Have More Fun* (New York: Harper Paperbacks, 2011).

Chapter 7. Permission to Prioritize Self-Care

1. Winifred A. Gebhardt and Stan Maes, "Competing Personal Goals and Exercise Behaviour," *Perceptual and Motor Skills* 86(3), June 1998, 755–759; Derek M. Griffith, Katie Gunter, and Julie Ober Allen, "Male Gender Role Strain as a Barrier to African American Men's Physical Activity," *Health Education & Behavior* 38(5), October 2011, 482–491.

2. Chloe E. Bird and Patricia P. Rieker, *Gender and Health: The Effects of Constrained Choices and Social Policies* (New York: Cambridge University Press, 2008); Julie Fleury, Colleen Keller, and Carolyn Murdaugh, "Social and Contextual Etiology of Coronary Heart Disease in Women," *Journal of Women's Health & Gender-Based Medicine* 9(9), November 2000, 967–978.

3. C. S. Mackenzie, W. L. Gekoski, and V. J. Knox, "Age, Gender, and the Underutilization of Mental Health Services: The Influence of Help-Seeking Attitudes," *Aging & Mental Health* 10(6), 2006, 574–582.

4. Michael E. Addis, *Invisible Men: Men's Inner Lives and the Consequences of Silence* (New York: Times Books, 2011), 8.
5. American Psychological Association, "Stress in America 2013 Highlights: Are Teens Adopting Adults' Stress Habits?" http://www.apa.org/news/press/releases/stress/2013/highlights.aspx. Accessed September 26, 2014.
6. Michael R. Irwin, "Why Sleep Is Important for Health: A Psychoneuroimmunology Perspective," *Annual Review of Psychology*, 2014.
7. Barbara L. Fredrickson and Christine Branigan, "Positive Emotions Broaden the Scope of Attention and Thought-Action Repertoires," *Cognition & Emotion* 19(3), 2005, 313–332.
8. Jacquelynne S. Eccles, "Subjective Task Value and the Eccles et al. Model of Achievement-Related Choices," in *Handbook of Competence and Motivation*, edited by Andrew J. Elliot and Carol S. Dweck (New York: Guilford Press, 2005), 105–121.
9. James N. Druckman and Arthur Lupia, "Preference Formation," *Annual Review of Political Science* 3, 2000, 1–24.
10. Carol S. Dweck, "Can Personality Be Changed? The Role of Beliefs in Personality and Change," *Current Directions in Psychological Science* 17(6), 2008, 391–394.
11. Druckman and Lupia, "Preference Formation," 5.
12. Norman Doidge, *The Brain That Changes Itself: Stories of Personal Triumph from the Frontiers of Brain Science* (New York: Penguin Books, 2007), xix.
13. Richard J. Davidson and Bruce S. McEwen, "Social Influences on Neuroplasticity: Stress and Interventions to Promote Well-Being," *Nature Neuroscience* 15, 2012, 689–695.
14. Ibid., 694.

Chapter 8. What Sustains Us, We Sustain

1. Arthur Lupia, "Communicating Science in Politicized Environments," *Proceedings of the National Academy of Sciences* 110 (Suppl. 3), August 20, 2013, 14048–14054.
2. Luke Wayne Henderson, Tess Knight, and Ben Richardson, "An Exploration of the Well-Being Benefits of Hedonic and Eudaimonic Behaviour," *Journal of Positive Psychology* 8(4), 2013, 322–336; Michelle L. Segar and Caroline R. Richardson, "Prescribing Pleasure and Meaning: Cultivating Walking Motivation and Maintenance," *American Journal of Preventive Medicine* 47(6), 2014, 838–841.
3. "Health," Online Etymology Dictionary, http://www.etymonline.com/index.php?term=health. Accessed September 25, 2014.
4. Jane Brody, "Changing America's Anthem on Exercise," *New York Times*, August 28, 2012, D7. http://well.blogs.nytimes.com/2012/08/27/changing-our-tune-on-exercise/.
5. Segar and Richardson, "Prescribing Pleasure and Meaning."
6. Henderson, Knight, and Richardson, "An Exploration of the Well-Being Benefits."
7. Barbara L. Fredrickson, "The Role of Positive Emotions in Positive Psychol-

ogy: The Broaden-and-Build Theory of Positive Emotions," *American Psychologist* 56(3), March 2001, 218–226.

8. Barbara L. Fredrickson, "Positive Emotions Broaden and Build," in *Advances in Experimental Social Psychology*, vol. 47, edited by Patricia Devine and Ashby Plant (San Diego, Calif.: Academic Press, 2013), 1–46; Lisa G. Aspinwall, "Rethinking the Role of Positive Affect in Self-Regulation," *Motivation and Emotion* 22(1), 1998, 1–17.

9. Fredrickson, "The Role of Positive Emotions."

10. Bethany E. Kok, Kimberly A. Coffey, Michael A. Cohn, Lahanna I. Catalino, Tanya Vacharkulksemsuk, Sara B. Algoe, Mary Brantley, and Barbara L. Frederickson, "How Positive Emotions Build Physical Health: Perceived Positive Social Connections Account for the Upward Spiral Between Positive Emotions and Vagal Tone," *Psychological Science* 24(7), July 2013, 1123–1132; Carol D. Ryff, "Eudaimonic Well-Being and Health: Mapping Consequences of Self-Realization," in *The Best Within Us: Positive Psychology Perspectives on Eudaimonia*, edited by Alan S. Waterman (Washington, D.C.: American Psychological Association, 2013), 77–98.

11. Henderson, Knight, and Richardson, "An Exploration of the Well-Being Benefits."

12. David A. Williams, David Kuper, Michelle L. Segar, Niveditha Mohan, Manish Sheth, and Daniel J. Clauw, "Internet-Enhanced Management of Fibromyalgia: A Randomized Controlled Trial," *Pain* 151(3), 2010, 694–702.

13. http://www.huffingtonpost.com/news/third-metric/.

Chapter 9. Six Big Ideas for Lifelong Sustainability

1. Carol S. Dweck, *Mindset: The New Psychology of Success* (New York: Ballantine Books, 2006).

2. Gary P. Latham and Edwin A. Locke, "New Developments in and Directions for Goal-Setting Research," *European Psychologist* 12(4), 2007, 290–300.

3. Ibid.

4. Paulo Freire, *Pedagogy of Indignation* (Boulder, Colo.: Paradigm, 2004), 15.

5. Paulo Freire, *Pedagogy of the Oppressed* (New York: Continuum, 1995).

Chapter 10. Sustainability Training

1. Shirli Kopelman, *Negotiating Genuinely: Being Yourself in Business* (Stanford, Calif.: Stanford University Press, 2014).

2. Esther K. Papies and Henk Aarts, "Nonconscious Self-Regulation, or the Automatic Pilot of Human Behavior," in *Handbook of Self-Regulation: Research, Theory, and Applications*, 2nd ed., edited by Kathleen D. Vohs and Roy F. Baumeister (New York: Guilford Press, 2011), 125–142.

3. Michelle L. Segar, Jacquelynne S. Eccles, and Caroline R. Richardson, "Type of Physical Activity Goal Influences Participation in Healthy Midlife Women," *Women's Health Issues* 18, 2008, 281–291.

4. Rafer S. Lutz, Paul Karoly, and Morris A. Okun, "The *Why* and the *How* of Goal Pursuit: Self-Determination, Goal Process Cognition, and Participation in Physical Exercise," *Psychology of Sport and Exercise* 9, 2008, 559–575.

5. Justin Presseau, Falko F. Sniehotta, Jill J. Francis, and Winifred A. Gebhardt, "With a Little Help from My Goals: Integrating Intergoal Facilitation with the Theory of Planned Behaviour to Predict Physical Activity," *British Journal of Health Psychology* 15(4), 2010, 905–919.

6. Maura L. Scott and Stephen M. Nowlis, "The Effect of Goal Specificity on Consumer Goal Reengagement," *Journal of Consumer Research* 40(3), 2013, 444–459.

7. Edward McAuley, Heidi-Mai Talbot, and Suzanne Martinez, "Manipulating Self-Efficacy in the Exercise Environment in Women: Influences on Affective Response," *Health Psychology* 18(3), May 1999, 288–294.

8. Inge Schweiger Gallo and Peter M. Gollwitzer, "Implementation Intentions: A Look Back at Fifteen Years of Progress, *Psicothema* 19(1), 2007, 37–42.

9. Ibid.

10. Ari Weinzweig, *A Lapsed Anarchist's Approach to Managing Ourselves* (Ann Arbor, Mich.: Zingerman's Press, 2013).

11. Cathy M. R. Magnus, Kent C. Kowalski, and Tara-Leigh F. McHugh, "The Role of Self-Compassion in Women's Self-Determined Motives to Exercise and Exercise-Related Outcomes," *Self and Identity* 9(4), 2010, 363–382; Leah J. Ferguson, Kent C. Kowalski, Diane E. Mack, and Catherine M. Sabiston, "Exploring Self-Compassion and Eudaimonic Well-Being in Young Women Athletes," *Journal of Sport & Exercise Psychology* 36(2), April 2014, 203–216.

12. Kristin Neff, *Self-Compassion: Stop Beating Yourself Up and Leave Insecurity Behind* (New York: HarperCollins, 2011).

13. Ibid.

Epilogue: Changing Your Beliefs, Changing Your Behavior, Changing Your Life

1. Carol S. Dweck, "Can Personality Be Changed?: The Role of Beliefs in Personality and Change," *Current Directions in Psychological Science* 17(6), 2008, 391–394.

2. Paulo Freire, *Pedagogy of the Oppressed* (New York: Continuum, 1995).

3. Edward L. Deci and Richard M. Ryan, *Intrinsic Motivation and Self-Determination in Human Behavior* (New York: Plenum Press, 1985).

4. Wijnand A. P. van Tilburg and Eric R. Igou, "On the Meaningfulness of Behavior: An Expectancy x Value Approach," *Motivation and Emotion* 37(3), September 2013, 373–388.

Index

About the Author

MICHELLE SEGAR IS A BEHAVIORAL SUSTAINABILITY AND MOTIVATION scientist and Director of the University of Michigan's Sport, Health, and Activity Research and Policy (SHARP) Center. She also chairs the U.S. National Physical Activity Plan's Communications Committee, advising the Plan on new strategies for the American public and policy makers. Her comprehensive training includes a Ph.D. in Psychology and master's degrees in Health Behavior/Health Education (MPH) and Kinesiology (MS) from the University of Michigan. Dr. Segar not only researches the science behind sustainable behavior change, she has learned first-hand how to put these theories to work, in real life, through her two decades of one-on-one health and well-being coaching with individuals.

Dr. Segar's broad base of experience has given her a unique 360-degree view of the most critical health issue facing our society: the failure to achieve widespread adoption of health-promoting and disease-management behaviors. Her approach to fitness, self-care, and health has gained the attention of both the media and influential members of the health field. Dr. Segar advises global organizations on the next-generation of communication strategies, counseling protocols, patient-centered systems, and app development to foster the engagement, commitment, and consistent decision making that underlie a lifetime of fitness, meaning, well-being, and health. She also delivers sustainable behavior change trainings to health professionals worldwide. Her ideas have generated accolades from such prestigious organizations as the Society of Behavioral Medicine, the Blue Cross Blue Shield of Michigan Foundation, and the North American Menopause Society, among others. Visit www.michellesegar.com.